THE BIG 10 PALEO SPIRALIZER COOKBOOK

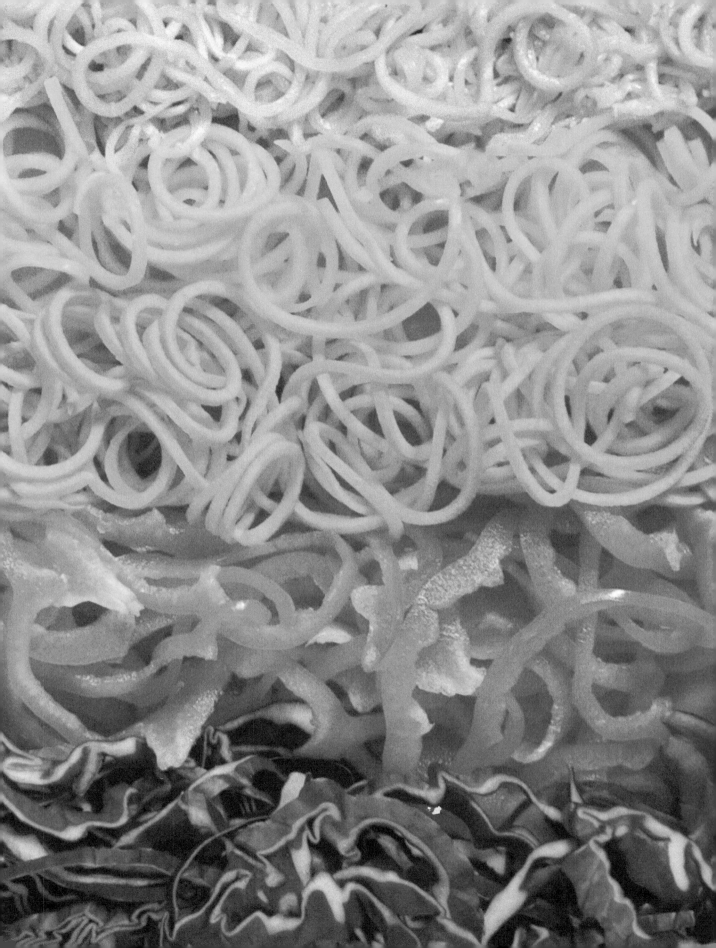

THE
BIG 10
PALEO
SPIRALIZER
COOKBOOK

10 VEGETABLES TO NOODLE, 100 HEALTHY SPIRALIZER RECIPES, 300 VARIATIONS

MEGAN FLYNN PETERSON

Photography by Shannon Douglas

ROCKRIDGE
PRESS

To Sean—my brother and my best friend

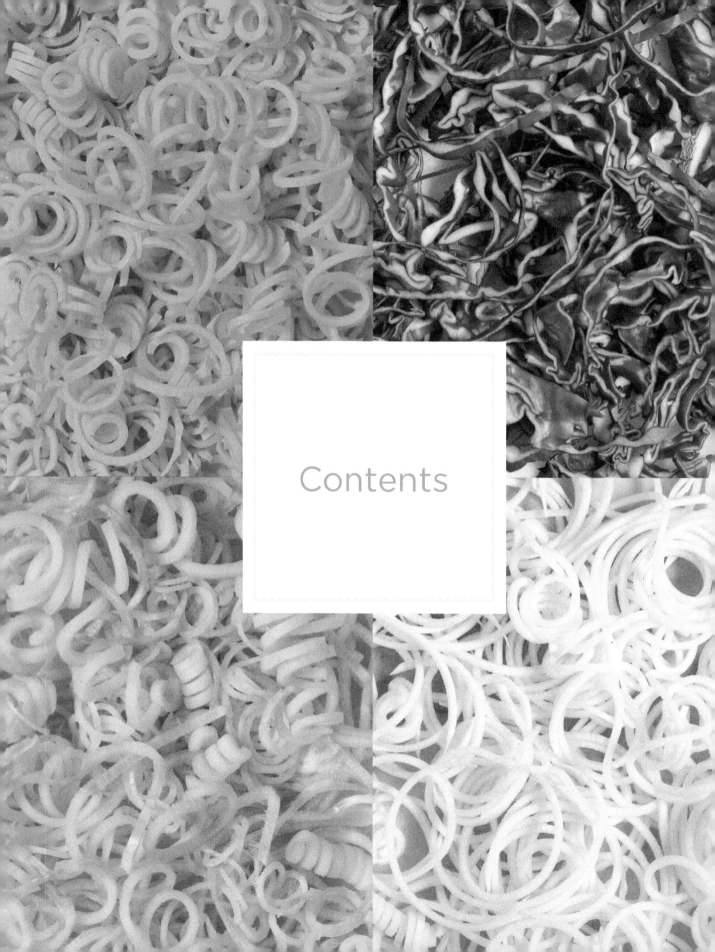

Contents

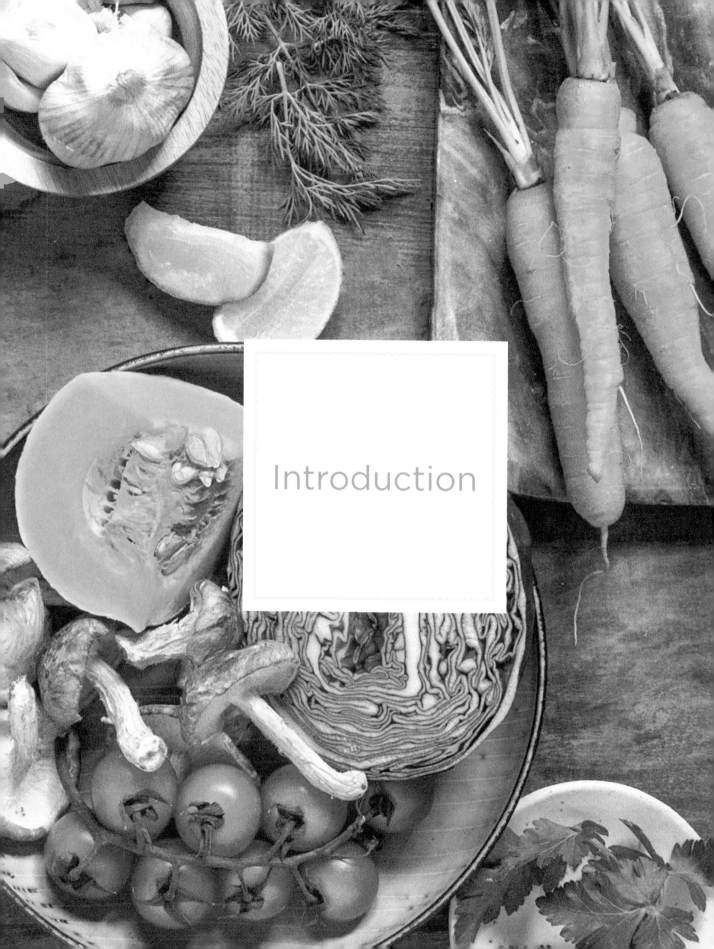

Introduction

I first discovered spiralizing about three years ago, but it wasn't spiralizing as I know it today. My mom used a julienne slicer to cut super-thin sheets of zucchini into lasagna-like sheets, and then she cut them into noodles with a knife. She threw them into a pan with olive oil and garlic, quickly sautéing them the way we used to do with spaghetti *aglio e olio* (or "emergency pasta," as we call it in my family).

We called them zucchini noodles, because that's what they were, but I don't think we had any idea just how many veggie-to-noodle options were out there. Then, a few years later, I got a handheld spiral veggie slicer; it was perfect for zucchini and carrots—really anything round, long, and skinny enough to fit. And finally, I upgraded the handheld spiralizer for an upright one, which opened a whole new world of spiralizing possibilities. My spiralizer now sits on my kitchen counter and gets used at least twice a week.

Spiralizing veggies and the Paleo diet go hand in hand for so many reasons, but the biggest one for me is that I miss pasta (and noodles in general). My mom's side of the family is Italian, and my brother and I grew up eating pasta all the time. Our favorite meals were pasta, with pesto, with tomato sauce, with meatballs—every way you can imagine it, we had it. These days, I'll occasionally have a cheat meal of rice noodles, such as takeout beef chow fun or chicken pad thai, and sometimes I'll even pick up gluten-free pasta from the grocery store when I'm really feeling that pasta craving, but it's nice to be able to stick to Paleo eating and make noodles out of veggies instead.

Spiralizing is a great way to experiment with different vegetables, as well. Turnips and daikon radishes are not usually vegetables I reach for at the market, but armed with my spiralizer, suddenly everything is a delicious experiment, and I can't wait to get new veggies back to my kitchen and see what kind of noodles they yield. You also get a lot "more" veggie when you spiralize it. As someone with a huge appetite, I really appreciate generous servings, especially when I'm trying to eat more reasonable portion sizes.

Whether you have serious feelings for noodles (as I do) or not, spiralizing is a great way to add some variety to your Paleo diet—and let's face it, the Paleo diet is great for your health, but it's easy to slowly but surely find yourself in a rut with the same old reliable meals. Spiralizing expands your culinary horizons and breaks you out of your routine. Between the different noodles you can make (ribbon noodles, fettuccini, spaghetti, etc.) and all the vegetables out there just waiting to be spiralized, there is no limit to flavor, texture, or variety. If you can peel it or slice it, chances are you can spiralize it.

Well, what are we waiting for? Let's get to it.

READY, SET, SPIRALIZE

Spiralizing is one of my favorite ways to eat vegetables. Who doesn't love a big bowl of noodles? I also think it's one of the easiest ways to prepare vegetables—you don't have to do any chopping or slicing, and the spiralizing itself is done in a flash.

While developing the recipes for this book, I had the best time coming up with dishes that are quick and easy but also flavorful and creative. I've loved being able to combine two of my food passions—the Paleo diet and noodles—to create this book.

Within these pages, you'll find breakfast dishes, dinners, light lunches, and creative and exciting snacks with plenty of variations that will ensure you never get bored of eating Paleo food. Several of the recipes are quick—most of them are 30 minutes and under, and those are labeled as such. You'll also find labels for dairy-free, nut-free, vegan, and raw recipes, but every recipe you encounter in the following chapters is 100 percent Paleo as well.

One of the things I love about spiralizing is how creative and fun it can be, so I hope you take these recipes and run with them—try them all, and then use your newfound knowledge to create your own fun, healthy, and colorful veggie noodle recipes.

WHY THIS BOOK

This book has a couple of goals: First and foremost, *The Big 10* aims to provide you with a wide variety of solid, delicious recipes for spiralized vegetables that will keep you excited about the Paleo diet, your spiralizer, and all that each has to offer. And I also want to uncover the wonderful, bonus result of spiralizing, which is being able to consistently feed yourself healthy meals without ever getting bored.

When your diet consists of the same old chicken, broccoli, and roasted sweet potatoes, it doesn't take long before you start craving new flavors and textures. Here you'll find innovative recipes and fun variations that will ensure that you don't ever have to make the same thing two nights in a row . . . unless you discover a favorite that you can't get enough of, in which case I say go for it!

You might notice that a few chapters have more recipes than others, which was done intentionally—zucchini and summer squash are extremely versatile and more commonly spiralized than, say, turnips. Although all of the vegetables in this book are delicious in their spiralized form, the longest chapter will focus on zucchini and summer squash.

Like in *The Big 15 Paleo Cookbook*, the variations you'll find after each recipe make it easy to throw together a great meal with whatever you have on hand, taking the stress out of meal planning and saving you those little one- or two-ingredient trips to the store. I want to encourage you to experiment—that's what's so great about veggie noodles! Once you learn how to prepare them, you can start getting creative when it comes to seasoning, sauces, protein pairings, and so much more.

THE GREAT SPIRALIZER CHEAT SHEET

One of my favorite things about spiralizing (and Paleo in general) is that you can cook a wide variety of dishes without ever really using a recipe. This little cheat sheet is here for those nights when you want to make something quick and healthy but don't have a ton of ingredients in your fridge. Do some mixing and matching and come up with something totally delicious and easy, every time.

NOODLES: ribbon noodles (blade A), fettuccini (blade B), linguini (blade C), or spaghetti (blade D).

VEGETABLES: zucchini, carrots, sweet potatoes, cucumber, butternut squash

PROTEIN: baked chicken, meatballs, grilled fish, Italian sausage, sliced pork

SAUCE: tomato sauce, pesto, creamy Alfredo (see page 28), balsamic vinaigrette, (see page 47) chili sesame vinaigrette

TOPPING: sliced olives, sliced green onion, sesame seeds, crushed almonds, fresh herbs

THE 10

As you've most likely already noticed, we're going to focus on 10 major vegetables in this book. Each chapter will give you the knowledge you'll need to spiralize and prepare the vegetable, followed by easy-to-prepare recipes. You'll also find two variations after each recipe, because I like options, and I think you will, too.

THE VEGGIES

These are the vegetables that make up the Big 10—they're the ones that stand up best to a spiralizer, and I think you'll find yourself spiralizing them again and again. In each chapter I'll let you know which blade on the spiralizer works best for each particular recipe, but all of the noodle shapes work well, so find your favorites and have fun with it.

- Zucchini and summer squash
- Beets
- Carrots
- Butternut squash
- Sweet potatoes

- Cucumbers
- Broccoli
- Turnips
- Cabbage
- Bell peppers

I personally use zucchini, carrots, and cucumbers the most, but all of the vegetables we'll be using yield gorgeous noodles, so try them all and discover your favorites.

The final chapter, "Pantry Basics," features five bonus recipes for homemade staples to use in your Paleo pantry, such as condiments, sauces, dressings, and quick pickles, all of which will enhance your kitchen repertoire and add an extra element of flavor to your favorite dishes.

BEYOND THE BASES

Here's a working list of some of the non-spiralized ingredients I use the most. The items listed here are those that appear most frequently in this book of recipes, so you can stock your kitchen and get cooking right away!

Proteins
Because the main ingredient of every recipe in this book is a vegetable, many of the recipes are vegetarian, or they can be made vegetarian easily. But another big part of the Paleo diet is meat, so we're going to be using a lot of the following proteins:

- Chicken
- Beef
- Pork

- Fish
- Shrimp
- Eggs

Herbs and Spices

I use fresh herbs as much as possible (usually rosemary, basil, sage, cilantro, thyme, and parsley), but it's great to keep dried herbs on hand as well for convenience and consistency, especially those that might not always be available fresh, such as thyme and oregano, and some that really come through in a pinch, like garlic powder.

- Cayenne pepper
- Chili seasoning
- Cumin, ground and seeds
- Curry powder
- Garlic powder
- Onion powder

- Oregano, dried
- Paprika, ground
- Red pepper flakes
- Taco seasoning (page 155)
- Thyme, ground

Other Vegetables

Some of the recipes will incorporate other veggies that aren't spiralized. Here's a good idea of what I usually have on hand to make many of the dishes you'll find in this book, as well as other everyday recipes I just kind of throw together.

- Onions (red and yellow—avoid sweet varieties)
- Celery
- Carrots (not just for spiralizing—they make a great aromatic beginning to most dishes)
- Tomatoes (fresh and canned—check canned tomato labels for added sugar)

- Spinach, kale, arugula, or salad mix (I like to keep a bag of one of these in my fridge and throw a handful into most dishes right before serving)
- Green onions
- Brussels sprouts
- Cauliflower

Pantry Items

In addition to fresh produce, meats, and spices, many of the recipes call for the pantry basics outlined here.

- Chili garlic oil or chili garlic sauce
- Ghee
- Grass-fed butter
- Olive oil, extra-virgin

- Paleo mayo (page 154)
- Nuts: almonds, cashews, pine nuts, pistachios, and walnuts
- Sesame oil

RECIPE LABELS

For your convenience, each recipe is paired with appropriate labels to help you decide what to make at a glance.

- **DF** Dairy-Free
- **NF** Nut-Free
- **R** Raw

- **30** 30 minutes or less
- **V** Vegan

BLADES OF GLORY

There are a few different kinds of spiralizers out there, and most of them will work well with the recipes in this book. It sounds silly, but my life has really changed since I bought a good spiralizer. Before, I was getting by with a handheld model or slicing noodles freestyle, with a knife, which was time-consuming and didn't offer much variety.

Choose a spiralizer with easy-to-change blades so you can switch up your noodles and keep food-related boredom at bay. They're generally labeled A, B, C, and D.

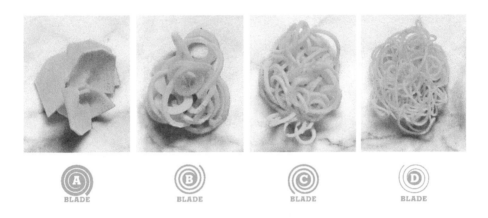

I use the Inspiralizer brand, but other great choices include Paderno, SpiraLife, Brieftons, and many more. The blades may differ in some ways, but overall, they have the same offerings. This is how we'll refer to them in this book:

Blade A: Ribbon Noodles—very wide and flat, 1/2" diameter
Blade B: Fettuccini—wide and flat, 1/4" diameter*
Blade C: Linguini—semi-wide and round, 1/4" diameter*
Blade D: Spaghetti—round and thin, 1/8" diameter

You may need to consult your manual to see which noodle and blade is which. A lot of the recipes, Creamy Fettuccini Alfredo (page 28) or Zucchini Spaghetti and Clams (page 33), for example, call for a specific noodle size, but I love experimenting with different shapes. For a long time, I thought blade D was my favorite, but now my go-to is blade C!

Keep in mind that noodles of different sizes will have different cooking times—ribbon noodles (A) will cook much more quickly than linguini (C) or spaghetti (D). You can pick a favorite and stick with it, but this book is going to have you switching it up a lot, and I encourage you to go with it!

Even though these blades are the same size, they create two distinct shapes that will cook quite differently!

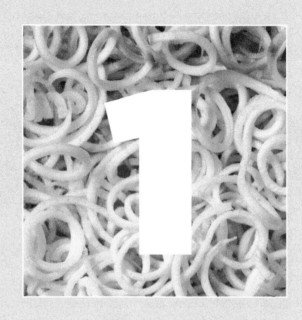

1
ZUCCHINI
AND SUMMER
SQUASH

Zucchini is the original vegetable for spiralizing, in my mind—they even have their own name! We call them zoodles instead of noodles. It was the first veggie noodle I ever encountered, and I think that's probably true for most people, so that's where we're going to start. In this chapter, you'll find 20 delicious zucchini and summer squash noodle recipes that are sure to make you miss conventional pasta a lot less. From fettuccini Alfredo to Cincinnati chili to Vietnamese pho soup, you'll be covered with this mammoth collection of zoodle and summer squash noodle recipes.

A lot of people swear by liberally salting their zucchini noodles and letting them "sweat" in a colander for 20 to 30 minutes before rinsing with water and gently drying with a towel. The point of this is to help them stay "al dente" in texture, closer to that of regular pasta. I agree that it helps keep them crunchy when you cook them, but I don't always do it—so if you have extra time, you can go for it, but none of the recipes I've written rely on this step to make or break them. Zucchini noodles take only a few minutes to cook, though, so you could always sweat them as you're making the rest of the dish—again, it's up to you.

ROASTED TOMATO *and* ZUCCHINI NOODLE FRITTATA

I love one-pan dishes a lot. Maybe it's because I'm lazy and don't want to have a lot to clean up, but a big part of it is that I think there is so much flavor when you cook everything in the same pan. This frittata is delicious and easy to make, and the addition of zucchini noodles ups the veggie content in an interesting and flavorful way. This is a go-to breakfast recipe in my house, especially if we're having guests. There's just something fancy about a frittata. **SERVES 2 TO 4**

PREP TIME: 10 minutes
COOK TIME: 30 minutes

DF **NF**

1 to 2 tablespoons extra-virgin olive oil

½ medium yellow onion, chopped

2 garlic cloves, minced

1 large zucchini, spiralized

Salt

Freshly ground black pepper

6 eggs

½ cup cherry tomatoes, halved

Sliced green onion, for garnish

PER SERVING Calories 174, Fat 14g, Protein 9g, Sodium 390mg, Total Carbs 5g, Fiber 1g

1. Preheat the oven to 350°F.

2. In a medium cast iron skillet over medium heat, heat the olive oil and sauté the onion and garlic until tender, about 5 minutes. Add the zucchini noodles and stir gently. Season with salt and pepper.

3. In a medium bowl, whisk the eggs.

4. Arrange the onion and the zucchini noodles so they're evenly spread out in the skillet. Slowly pour the eggs in and increase the heat to medium-high. Season with salt and pepper and allow to cook until the edges start to pull away from the skillet, 3 to 4 minutes.

5. Add the cherry tomatoes to the skillet and transfer to the oven. Cook until the top is no longer runny, 15 to 20 minutes.

6. Remove from the oven, allow to cool slightly, and serve garnished with sliced green onion.

VARIATION 1 **BLT ZUCCHINI NOODLE FRITTATA:** Add 3 or 4 slices chopped bacon to the skillet (eliminate the olive oil) and sauté with the onions and garlic. Follow the rest of the original recipe as written. Top the sliced frittata with a handful of chopped lettuce instead of green onion. (You could even add a drizzle of Paleo Ranch Dressing—page 154.)

VARIATION 2 **PIZZA FRITTATA:** Add ½ cup chopped pepperoni to the onion, garlic, and zucchini. Follow the rest of the original recipe and serve with a side of pizza sauce (just make sure there's no added sugar).

SUMMER SQUASH NOODLE SALAD
with **TOMATO** and **AVOCADO**

 This salad is perfect for spring and summer—the zucchini noodles are raw, so everything is super crunchy and fresh. If you've been salting your squash noodles before cooking up until this point, now is a good time to skip it. Just give the summer squash a rinse before spiralizing, and it'll be ready to go! I love the addition of balsamic vinaigrette to these vegetables, but you could mix it up however you like (I've included one idea in the first variation)! **SERVES 4 TO 6**

PREP TIME: 20 minutes

4 or 5 summer squash, spiralized

1 cup cherry tomatoes, sliced

2 avocados, diced

½ cup extra-virgin olive oil

¼ cup balsamic vinegar

1 tablespoon Dijon mustard

1 garlic clove, minced

Salt

Freshly ground black pepper

PER SERVING Calories 317
Fat 30g, Protein 4g, Sodium 246mg,
Total Carbs 13g, Fiber 7g

1. In a large bowl, mix to combine the squash noodles with the cherry tomatoes and avocado.

2. In a small bowl, whisk together the olive oil, balsamic vinegar, Dijon mustard, and garlic. Season with salt and pepper and drizzle over the salad. Toss to combine and serve immediately.

VARIATION 1 **SUMMER SQUASH NOODLE SALAD WITH CILANTRO-LIME DRESSING:** Instead of balsamic vinaigrette, toss this salad in a cilantro-lime dressing: Mix ½ cup extra-virgin olive oil with ¼ cup freshly squeezed lime juice and 2 to 3 tablespoons chopped fresh cilantro.

VARIATION 2 **SUMMER SQUASH SALAD WITH GREENS:** Skip the tomatoes and add 1 to 2 cups fresh arugula or spinach (or a mix) to this salad. Top with ¼ cup sliced almonds.

ZUCCHINI RIBBON SALAD with PINE NUTS and BASIL

This salad is kind of a deconstructed pesto dish—I've always loved that pesto is a raw sauce. The zucchini noodles for this dish are cut in ribbons, and we're going to dress it with olive oil, a little bit of garlic, some toasted pine nuts, and plenty of fresh basil. It's delicious any time of year, but especially in the warmer months. **SERVES 4 TO 6**

PREP TIME: 15 minutes
COOK TIME: 5 minutes, plus 10 to 15 minutes to rest

3 or 4 large zucchini, spiralized

½ cup extra-virgin olive oil

2 garlic cloves, minced

¼ cup pine nuts

1½ cups lightly packed fresh basil, chopped

Salt

Freshly ground black pepper

PER SERVING Calories 206 Fat 21g, Protein 3g, Sodium 207mg, Total Carbs 6g, Fiber 2g

1. Place the zucchini noodles in a large bowl.

2. In a small bowl, mix to combine the olive oil and garlic.

3. In a small, dry pan over medium-low heat, toast the pine nuts, stirring frequently until fragrant, about 3 minutes, and quickly remove from the heat. Add them to the zucchini noodles and toss to combine. Dress the salad with the garlicky olive oil. Toss again.

4. Add the chopped basil to the salad and toss to combine. Season with salt and pepper. Allow to rest for 10 to 15 minutes (more if possible) before serving.

VARIATION 1 CHICKEN ZUCCHINI RIBBON SALAD WITH PINE NUTS AND BASIL: Serve this salad topped with ½ pound grilled chicken breast slices. To grill the chicken, brush with olive oil and season with salt and pepper. Cook on a grill or grill pan over medium heat for 8 to 10 minutes per side, until completely opaque and the juices run clear.

VARIATION 2 ZUCCHINI RIBBON SALAD WITH LEMON AND DILL: Dress the zucchini noodles with garlic olive oil as directed in original recipe, omit the basil, and add the juice of 1 lemon and 2 tablespoons fresh chopped dill. Season with salt and pepper. Toss to combine and allow to rest for 10 to 15 minutes before serving.

"TORTELLINI" SOUP

  Sometimes I wonder if my perception of "comfort food" is skewed because I ate so much pasta as a kid. I don't really remember eating chicken noodle soup when I was sick, but my mom would pour chicken broth over tortellini and top it with so much delicious, salty Parmesan cheese that it would sink to the bottom of my mug and get stuck on the back of my spoon. This "tortellini" soup is actually missing the tortellini, since cheese isn't Paleo, but the little summer squash knots are super cute, and the broth is just as good as it always was. **SERVES 2 TO 4**

PREP TIME: 15 minutes
COOK TIME: 15 minutes

NF 30

2 tablespoons grass-fed butter

1 medium yellow onion, diced

2 garlic cloves, minced

2 medium celery stalks, diced

1 large carrot, chopped

Salt

Freshly ground black pepper

4 cups chicken (or beef) broth

4 summer squash, spiralized

PER SERVING Calories 142
Fat 8g, Protein 8g, Sodium 1,133mg,
Total Carbs 12g, Fiber 3g

1. In a large pot over medium heat, melt the butter. Sauté the onion and garlic until the onion is tender, 5 to 7 minutes, or until the veggies become fork-tender.

2. Add the celery and carrot and cook for another 5 to 7 minutes. Season with salt and pepper. Pour the chicken broth over the vegetables and stir. Bring to a simmer.

3. While the broth is boiling, cut your squash noodles into 3-inch pieces. Tie each one into a knot (to resemble a tortellini). Gently lower the squash noodle tortellini into the broth and cook for 2 to 3 minutes. Don't fret if a few of them open up.

4. Ladle the soup into bowls and enjoy hot.

VARIATION 1 VEGETARIAN "TORTELLINI" SOUP: Make this soup vegetarian by using veggie broth instead of chicken broth.

VARIATION 2 "TORTELLINI" SOUP WITH CHICKEN: After adding the broth to the pot, add 1 diced boneless chicken breast to the pot. Cook until the meat is completely opaque, 8 to 10 minutes. Follow the remaining original recipe steps as listed.

ZUCCHINI NOODLE PHO

One of my all-time favorite things to eat on a chilly afternoon is a big, hot bowl of pho. My friend Corri and I used to meet at different Vietnamese restaurants and chow down on rice noodles, deliciously savory broth, and all the fresh toppings like bean sprouts, jalapeños, and basil leaves. My mouth is watering just thinking about it! I wanted to include a Paleo recipe for pho so I wouldn't always be relying on takeout (and rice noodles) to satisfy my craving. **SERVES 2 TO 4**

PREP TIME: 15 minutes
COOK TIME: 6 hours, 40 minutes

About 4 pounds beef soup bones

1 medium yellow onion, halved

2 garlic cloves, sliced

2 or 3 star anise pods

2 to 3 tablespoons peeled, sliced fresh ginger

2 to 3 tablespoons fish sauce

Salt

Freshly ground black pepper

4 quarts water

1 to 2 pounds beef sirloin, sliced very thin

2 or 3 large zucchini, spiralized

TOPPINGS FOR SOUP

chopped fresh cilantro, sliced green onion, bean sprouts, chopped fresh Thai (or regular) basil, lime wedges, chili garlic oil or chili garlic sauce

PER SERVING Calories 499
Fat 15g, Protein 75g, Sodium 1,500, Total Carbs 11g, Fiber 3g

1. Preheat the oven to 400°F.

2. Spread the bones and onion out on a large baking pan and roast for 40 minutes to 1 hour. (This step is optional but really brings out a lot of the flavor in the beef broth.)

3. Put the bones and onion in a large stock pot with the garlic, star anise, ginger, fish sauce, and some salt and pepper. Cover everything with the water and bring to a boil. Reduce the heat to low and allow the pot to simmer for at least 6 hours, or up to 24 hours. Strain the broth and use immediately, or refrigerate until ready to serve.

4. Bring the broth to a simmer and add the sliced beef. While the beef is cooking, divide the zucchini noodles among 2 to 4 serving bowls. Once the beef is pink (should take 5 to 7 minutes), spoon broth over the noodles and top the soup with cooked beef. Add cilantro, green onion, bean sprouts, basil, lime, and chili garlic oil as desired and serve.

VARIATION 1 QUICKER PHO: Use store-bought beef broth if you don't have time to make the broth yourself—just quickly char the onion, garlic, and other spices in a dry skillet before transferring to a large pot. Pour the beef broth overtop and bring everything to a simmer. Strain the broth and proceed as directed in the original recipe.

VARIATION 2 ZUCCHINI NOODLE PHO WITH MUSHROOMS AND BOK CHOY: Add 10 ounces sliced mushrooms and 1½ cups baby bok choy to the broth. Follow the remaining recipe as written.

EASY SESAME NOODLES

 This is one of my all-time favorite recipes. Before my Paleo days, I'd whip this up with regular old spaghetti and it was always so good. The sauce is more of a dressing than anything else, and all you have to do is quickly pan-fry the zucchini noodles before tossing it all together. There's just something about hot, fresh sesame noodles served straight out of the pan that really speaks to me. **SERVES 2 TO 4**

PREP TIME: 10 minutes
COOK TIME: 5 minutes

1 to 2 tablespoons extra-virgin olive oil

2 or 3 garlic cloves, minced

2 or 3 large zucchini or summer squash, spiralized

¼ cup coconut aminos

2 tablespoons rice vinegar

3 to 4 tablespoons sesame oil

½ teaspoon chili garlic oil

Salt, if needed

Freshly ground black pepper, if needed

Sliced green onion, for garnish

PER SERVING Calories 234
Fat 22g, Protein 2g, Sodium 266mg,
Total Carbs 9g, Fiber 2g

1. In a large skillet over medium heat, heat the olive oil and sauté the garlic for 1 to 2 minutes. Add the zucchini noodles and sauté for 3 to 4 minutes or until the noodles start to become fork-tender. Remove from the heat.

2. While the noodles are cooking, mix the coconut aminos, rice vinegar, sesame oil, and chili garlic oil together. Taste and season with salt and pepper if necessary.

3. Transfer the noodles to a large bowl, pour the sesame sauce over them, and toss to combine. Serve garnished with sliced green onion.

VARIATION 1 **PORK BELLY SESAME NOODLES:** Instead of using olive oil, pan-fry about ½ pound diced pork belly over medium-high heat for 4 to 5 minutes, until crispy and browned, before adding the garlic. Follow the remaining recipe steps as written. (If you can't find pork belly, use pork loin marinated in some extra chili garlic oil.)

VARIATION 2 **SESAME NOODLES WITH KIMCHI:** Top this recipe with as much Kimchi Cabbage Noodles (page 138) as you'd like.

DRUNKEN ZUCCHINI NOODLES

 I included a Paleo pad thai recipe in my first book, so this time I wanted to share with you my drunken noodles, which always remind me of my best friend, Tina. She and I always eat Thai food whenever we're together—it's kind of our go-to, and neither of us can get enough of it (something our husbands both find a bit tedious). This recipe skips the rice noodles in exchange for zucchini ones, but it has all the spicy, delicious flavor of the original. **SERVES 2**

PREP TIME: 10 minutes
COOK TIME: 15 minutes

2 tablespoons extra-virgin olive oil

3 garlic cloves, minced

1 or 2 Thai chiles, seeded and chopped (depending on how spicy you like it)

2 or 3 green onions, finely chopped

¼ cup green bell pepper, sliced thin

3 tablespoons coconut aminos

2 tablespoons fish sauce

1 teaspoon honey (optional)

2 or 3 large zucchini, spiralized

2 or 3 plum tomatoes, chopped

1 cup lightly packed fresh basil leaves, chopped

Lime wedges, for garnish

PER SERVING Calories 246 Fat 15g, Protein 7g, Sodium 1,442mg, Total Carbs 27g, Fiber 6g

1. In a large skillet over medium heat, heat the olive oil and sauté the garlic until fragrant, about 1 minute. Add the chiles, green onions, and bell pepper. Give it a stir and cook until the vegetables are tender, about 5 minutes.

2. Add the coconut aminos, fish sauce, and honey (if using) to the skillet. Stir until combined. Add the zucchini noodles and tomatoes, stirring until everything is coated in sauce and the noodles are done, about 5 minutes.

3. Turn off the heat and stir in the chopped basil leaves. Serve immediately with the lime wedges.

VARIATION 1 CHICKEN AND SHRIMP DRUNKEN NOODLES: Sauté ½ pound diced chicken and ½ pound shrimp in the pan with the garlic. (The chicken should be cooked through in about 7 to 8 minutes, and you can add the shrimp about halfway through that cooking time, remembering to flip the shrimp after 2 minutes.) Add the rest of the veggies and follow the original recipe—you may need to add a bit more coconut aminos and fish sauce, depending on how saucy you like your dish.

VARIATION 2 SPICY BEEF DRUNKEN NOODLES: Thinly slice a sirloin steak and marinate it with coconut aminos and a teaspoon of crushed red pepper for 20 minutes. Sauté the meat with the garlic and other veggies. Follow the rest of the original recipe as written.

BEEF CHOW FUN

   Beef chow fun is my most recent favorite Chinese dish—I love the wide, flat noodles that are almost slippery against my rough chopsticks. It's a little bit like lo mein, but chow fun uses rice noodles instead of wheat ones, which is how I started ordering it soon after my husband and I moved to California from North Carolina. We've moved quite a few times, and we always say it's not home until you have a Chinese takeout place. This Paleo beef chow fun uses zucchini fettuccini noodles instead of rice noodles, and you can make it at home no matter where you live. **SERVES 2 TO 4**

PREP TIME: 10 minutes
COOK TIME: 15 minutes

DF **NF** **30**

3 tablespoons extra-virgin olive oil, divided

8 ounces flank steak, sliced thin

3 garlic cloves, minced

1 tablespoon peeled fresh ginger, sliced thin

4 or 5 green onions, chopped

2 or 3 heads baby bok choy, quartered

2 or 3 large zucchini, spiralized

1 tablespoon rice vinegar

3 to 4 tablespoons coconut aminos

4 to 6 ounces bean sprouts (omit if strict Paleo)

Salt (if needed)

Freshly ground black pepper (if needed)

PER SERVING Calories 279 Fat 16g, Protein 22g, Sodium 996mg, Total Carbs 15g, Fiber 4g

1. In a large skillet over medium-high heat, heat 1 tablespoon of the olive oil. Add the steak and cook until browned, about 5 minutes. Remove from the skillet and set aside.

2. Lower the heat to medium and add the remaining 2 tablespoons of olive oil. Stir in the garlic and ginger and allow to cook for about 1 minute. Add the green onions and bok choy and cook for another 2 to 3 minutes.

3. Add the zucchini noodles to the pan and stir. Pour in the rice vinegar and coconut aminos and toss to combine. Add the bean sprouts and allow everything to cook together until the zucchini noodles are tender, 3 to 4 minutes. Return the beef to the skillet to reheat, 1 to 2 minutes before serving.

4. Season with salt and pepper, if necessary, and serve hot.

VARIATION 1 CHICKEN CHOW FUN: Instead of beef, use 8 ounces sliced boneless chicken breast. Follow the recipe as written, but allow extra cooking time (just a few more minutes) for the chicken to become completely opaque.

VARIATION 2 VEGGIE CHOW FUN (WITH EGG): Skip the meat and add 2 spiralized or julienned carrots and 1 sliced red bell pepper to the skillet with the garlic and ginger. Before serving, either move all the ingredients to the side and scramble an egg in the open space of the pan, incorporating it into the rest of the ingredients, or plate the dish, fry a few eggs in the pan, and top each serving with a fried egg.

CREAMY FETTUCCINI ALFREDO

BLADE I know what you're thinking: How can a cream sauce like Alfredo be made Paleo? I used to wonder the same thing, until I discovered the magical creamy properties that cashews have. Making the sauce itself is quicker than it seems—if you soak the cashews overnight and roast the garlic ahead of time, all you have to do is throw everything into the food processor or blender and serve. Plan ahead a bit and enjoy this super-easy Paleo fettuccini Alfredo! **SERVES 4**

PREP TIME: 10 minutes, plus 6 hours or overnight to soak
COOK TIME: 45 minutes

2 cups raw cashews

1 large head garlic

1 tablespoon extra-virgin olive oil

1 tablespoon grass-fed butter

¼ cup minced shallot

1½ to 2 cups coconut or almond milk

Salt

Freshly ground black pepper

4 large zucchini, spiralized

PER SERVING Calories 777 Fat 67g, Protein 17g, Sodium 306mg, Total Carbs 40g, Fiber 7g

1. In a large bowl, cover the cashews with water and soak for at least 6 hours. You can do this overnight so they're ready when you are.

2. Preheat the oven to 350°F.

3. Cut off and discard the top of the head of garlic, place the garlic on a baking sheet, and drizzle with the olive oil. Wrap in foil and bake for about 40 minutes, until golden and the cloves in the center pierce easily with a knife.

4. A few minutes before the garlic is done roasting, in a large skillet over medium heat, melt the butter and sauté the shallot until translucent, about 4 minutes. Set the skillet aside.

5. Put the drained cashews in a food processor with the roasted garlic—just pop the cloves out of the skin. Add the sautéed shallot and 1½ cups of the coconut milk and blend. Adjust the amount of coconut milk depending on how thin or thick you like your sauce. Season with salt and pepper.

6. In the skillet you used for the shallot, over medium-high heat, quickly sauté the zucchini noodles until fork-tender, 3 to 4 minutes. Season with salt and pepper.

7. Add as much sauce as desired, mix well, and serve warm.

VARIATION 1 CHICKEN ALFREDO: While the garlic is roasting, sauté 1 pound diced chicken in a skillet over medium heat with about 1 tablespoon olive oil until cooked through, 7 to 8 minutes. Add the cooked chicken to the zucchini noodles and sauce before serving.

VARIATION 2 FETTUCCINI ALFREDO WITH SHRIMP: Sauté 1 pound shrimp in a skillet over medium heat with 1 tablespoon olive oil, an extra clove of minced garlic, and a squeeze of fresh lemon juice, about 2 minutes per side. Top the zucchini fettuccini Alfredo with shrimp and garnish with 1 tablespoon chopped fresh parsley before serving.

FETTUCCINI BOLOGNESE

BLADE When I think about Italian comfort food, hearty meat and tomato sauce comes to mind. Sure, spaghetti and meatballs are great, but there's just something about a thick sauce where everything is incorporated already. You won't miss the cream in this rich Paleo take on classic Bolognese! **SERVES 2 TO 4**

PREP TIME: 10 minutes
COOK TIME: 30 minutes

3 tablespoons grass-fed butter or extra-virgin olive oil

1 medium yellow onion, chopped

2 or 3 garlic cloves, minced

2 or 3 celery stalks, chopped

2 to 4 carrots, chopped

1 pound ground beef (preferably grass-fed)

Salt

Freshly ground black pepper

1 (28-ounce) can crushed tomatoes (no sugar added)

3 or 4 large zucchini, spiralized

PER SERVING Calories 439
Fat 16g, Protein 43g, Sodium 881mg,
Total Carbs 32g, Fiber 11g

1. In a large saucepan over medium heat, melt the butter. Sauté the onion, stirring regularly, until it becomes translucent and starts to caramelize, 8 to 10 minutes. Add the garlic and stir well before adding the celery and carrot. Cook another 5 to 7 minutes or until the veggies become fork-tender.

2. Move the sautéed vegetables to the edges of the pot, opening up a space in the center. Put the ground beef in the center of the pot and mix it up as it begins to brown. After a few minutes, start incorporating the vegetables into the beef and stir everything together. Season with salt and pepper.

3. Pour the crushed tomatoes into the pot, give it a stir, and bring the whole thing to a simmer before reducing the heat to low. Fill the tomato can halfway with water, and pour it into the pot. Stir again and reduce, cooking down the amount of liquid, for 10 to 15 minutes. If the sauce seems too thick, add more water.

4. In a large skillet over medium heat, sauté the zucchini fettuccini for 3 to 4 minutes, or until tender. Season with salt and pepper.

5. Transfer the noodles to plates or bowls, spoon the Bolognese overtop, and serve.

VARIATION 1 PANCETTA BOLOGNESE: Add about 4 ounces diced pancetta to the pot with the onion and garlic. Follow steps 3 to 5 of the recipe as written.

VARIATION 2 MUSHROOM BOLOGNESE: Add 10 ounces sliced mushrooms to the pot with the onion. Sauté until they begin to get brown and crispy, 7 to 8 minutes, and then add the rest of the veggies, followed by the beef, and finish the recipe as written.

GUILTLESS SPAGHETTI CARBONARA

   Is there anything more comforting or indulgent than spaghetti carbonara? I really don't think so. This creamy, egg yolk–based sauce is loaded with pancetta for a beautiful depth of flavor. Coconut cream makes this Paleo version dairy-free, but it keeps the fat content nice and high so you get a truly luxurious dish. This is one of my favorite dishes to make for friends—it's super easy to throw together, but it's impressive to serve, so I like that it's as special as it is delicious. **SERVES 2 TO 4**

PREP TIME: 10 minutes
COOK TIME: 20 minutes

DF **NF** **30**

6 to 8 ounces diced pancetta

½ medium yellow onion, diced

2 garlic cloves, minced

2 or 3 large zucchini, spiralized

Salt

Freshly ground black pepper

1 to 2 tablespoons coconut cream

1 egg plus 1 egg yolk

Fresh parsley, for garnish

PER SERVING Calories 402
Fat 30g, Protein 25g, Sodium 1,636mg,
Total Carbs 9g, Fiber 2g

1. In a large skillet over medium-high heat, cook the pancetta until it begins to crisp, about 5 minutes. Use a slotted spoon to transfer the pancetta to a paper towel-lined plate. Add the onion and garlic to the skillet and cook until golden, stirring frequently, about 5 minutes.

2. Add the zucchini noodles to the skillet and sauté until tender, about 5 minutes. Season with salt and pepper and reduce the heat to low.

3. In a small bowl, whisk the coconut cream, whole egg, and egg yolk. Season with salt and pepper.

4. Slowly pour the egg mixture over the zucchini noodles, mixing or tossing constantly with a spoon or tongs. (You want the mixture to become a creamy sauce that coats the noodles without the eggs scrambling.)

5. To serve, transfer the zucchini noodles to bowls or plates and top with pancetta and a sprinkle of fresh parsley.

VARIATION 1 SPAGHETTI CARBONARA WITH PEAS: Add ½ cup green peas (thawed if frozen) to the skillet with the zucchini noodles. Follow the rest of the recipe as written.

VARIATION 2 SPAGHETTI CARBONARA WITH CHICKEN: For an additional boost of protein, add about 1 pound diced boneless chicken breast to the skillet with the onions and pancetta. Cook, stirring frequently, until the chicken is cooked through and the onions are golden, 6 to 8 minutes, and then follow the remaining steps of the recipe as written.

ZOODLES with MARINATED OLIVES and ARTICHOKES

  This is one of those dishes that you put together one night because the ingredients are all randomly in your refrigerator and pantry, and before you know it you're putting them on your shopping list so you can make it again and again. Zucchini noodles with olives, a bit of citrus, and artichokes come together for a dish so fresh and delicious that I bet it'll become a regular occurrence in your meal-planning repertoire. Experiment with different olives in this dish, or use your favorites—I absolutely love Kalamata and Castelvetrano olives. **SERVES 2 TO 4**

PREP TIME: 10 minutes, plus several hours or overnight to marinate

COOK TIME: 10 minutes

½ cup pitted black olives (such as Kalamata)

½ cup pitted green olives (such as Castelvetrano)

½ cup extra-virgin olive oil, plus more for sautéing

Juice and zest of 1 lemon

1 garlic clove, minced

2 or 3 tablespoons chopped fresh basil, plus 1 tablespoon for garnish

Salt

Freshly ground black pepper

2 or 3 large zucchini, spiralized

1 (14-ounce) can artichoke hearts, drained

PER SERVING Calories 331 Fat 30g, Protein 6g, Sodium 692mg, Total Carbs 19g, Fiber 9g

1. Place the olives in a container with a lid. Add the olive oil, lemon juice and zest, garlic, and basil. Season with salt and pepper and mix well. Cover and refrigerate for several hours (overnight if possible). Remove from the refrigerator and allow to come to room temperature.

2. In a large skillet over medium heat, sauté the zucchini noodles in olive oil for about 5 minutes. Season with salt and pepper. Add the drained artichokes to the skillet. Once the artichokes are hot, after about 5 minutes, reduce the heat to low and add the olives and their marinade. Mix well to combine, adding more olive oil if necessary.

3. Serve immediately with more chopped basil.

VARIATION 1 GRILLED SALMON ZOODLES WITH MARINATED OLIVES AND ARTICHOKES: Add a 4- to 6-ounce piece of grilled salmon to each serving of the original recipe—to cook salmon, coat the salmon with a drizzle of olive oil and season with salt and pepper. Use a grill or grill pan to cook over medium heat for 3 to 5 minutes per side, until it flakes easily with a fork.

VARIATION 2 ZOODLES WITH CAPERS AND ARTICHOKES: For a nice salty bite without having to take the time to marinate the olives, omit the marinated olives and add about ½ cup drained capers to the skillet with the artichokes.

ZUCCHINI SPAGHETTI and CLAMS

 This is a recipe my family has enjoyed for as long as I can remember—I have vivid memories of my mom whipping it up and my dad being really excited about it every time. As a kid, I wasn't super enthusiastic about clams, but now I love them. We usually use canned clams (including the juice) for this recipe, but if you wanted to fancy it up a bit, you could use fresh ones in the shell—just make sure you discard any that don't open after cooking. Clams, garlic, and olive oil are so lovely together that no one will know you threw it all together in well under 30 minutes. **SERVES 4**

PREP TIME: 10 minutes
COOK TIME: 5 minutes

DF **NF** **30**

2 tablespoons extra-virgin olive oil

2 garlic cloves, minced

1 or 2 (6.5-ounce) cans clams with juice

3 or 4 large zucchini, spiralized

Salt

Freshly ground black pepper

¼ to ½ teaspoon crushed red pepper

3 or 4 green onions, finely chopped

Fresh parsley, chopped, for garnish

PER SERVING Calories 143
Fat 8g, Protein 3g, Sodium 647mg,
Total Carbs 18g, Fiber 3g

1. In a large skillet over medium heat, heat the olive oil and sauté the garlic for about 1 minute. Add the clams with their juice and give it a stir.

2. Add the zucchini noodles and sauté until tender, about 5 minutes. Gently stir to combine all ingredients. Season with salt and pepper and add the crushed red pepper. Remove from the heat and add the sliced green onions.

3. Serve hot with a sprinkle of chopped fresh parsley.

VARIATION 1 ZUCCHINI SPAGHETTI AND CLAMS WITH FRESH TOMATO: Add 1 cup of diced fresh tomato to the skillet before serving. (Stir for 1 to 2 minutes so they heat up a bit.)

VARIATION 2 LEMON-BUTTER ZUCCHINI SPAGHETTI WITH CLAMS: Instead of olive oil, sauté the garlic in 2 to 3 tablespoons grass-fed butter. Squeeze ½ lemon in the skillet before adding the clams and zucchini noodles. Follow the rest of the recipe as written, but garnish with a lemon wedge as well as the fresh parsley.

PASTA PRIMAVERA

    This dish is so delicious, and I love how loaded with vegetables it is! This recipe is a great way to get rid of any vegetables that need to be eaten, and you can definitely experiment and add whatever you'd like to it, but this is my go-to "default" primavera, if you will. **SERVES 6**

PREP TIME: 15 minutes
COOK TIME: 10 minutes

DF NF V 30

¼ cup extra-virgin olive oil

4 garlic cloves, sliced thin

1 large zucchini, spiralized

2 yellow squash, spiralized

Salt

Freshly ground black pepper

3 carrots, spiralized (or cut into thin pieces)

1 red bell pepper, cut into thin strips

½ cup broccoli florets

½ cup cherry tomatoes, halved

¼ teaspoon crushed red pepper

½ cup fresh basil, chopped

PER SERVING Calories 115
Fat 9g, Protein 2g, Sodium 229mg,
Total Carbs 10g, Fiber 3g

1. In a large skillet over medium heat, heat the olive oil and sauté the garlic for 1 minute or so, or until fragrant. Add the zucchini and yellow squash noodles and stir gently. Allow to cook for 3 to 4 minutes, or until the noodles start to become fork-tender. Season with salt and pepper.

2. Add the carrots, bell pepper, broccoli, and cherry tomatoes. Toss everything together and cook for another 3 to 4 minutes. Season again with salt and pepper, this time adding the crushed red pepper.

3. Remove from the heat, add the basil, toss one last time, and serve.

VARIATION 1 **CHICKEN PASTA PRIMAVERA:** Add about 1 pound cooked, diced boneless chicken to the skillet when you add the additional veggies in step two.

VARIATION 2 **ALFREDO PRIMAVERA:** Use cashew Alfredo sauce (page 28), adding ¼ to ½ cup, depending on how saucy you like your pasta.

SPIRALIZED RATATOUILLE

 I like ratatouille a lot, but sometimes there's something about the texture of a bunch of sautéed vegetables all cooked together that feels a little boring to me. This spiralized ratatouille incorporates zucchini, squash, and bell pepper noodles with diced eggplant and cherry tomatoes to give you some variety in the texture of this otherwise classic recipe. You could even spiralize the onion if you wanted—it's a lot faster and makes for a great presentation. **SERVES 6**

PREP TIME: 20 minutes
COOK TIME: 20 minutes

DF **NF** **V**

¼ cup extra-virgin olive oil

1 medium yellow onion, diced or spiralized

2 garlic cloves, minced

1 medium eggplant, diced

1 green bell pepper, spiralized

1 red bell pepper, spiralized

2 large zucchini, spiralized

2 or 3 summer squash, spiralized

1½ cups cherry tomatoes, halved

Salt

Freshly ground black pepper

½ teaspoon fresh thyme

1 tablespoon chopped fresh basil

PER SERVING Calories 147
Fat 9g, Protein 4g, Sodium 216mg,
Total Carbs 17g, Fiber 6g

1. In a large skillet over medium heat, heat the olive oil and sauté the onion. After 2 to 3 minutes, add the garlic. Give it a stir and add the eggplant. Cook, stirring frequently, until the eggplant is tender, 8 to 10 minutes.

2. Add the bell peppers, zucchini, summer squash, and cherry tomatoes and season with salt and pepper. Add the thyme and continue to cook for another 5 minutes.

3. Remove from the heat and add the basil, tossing to combine. Serve hot.

VARIATION 1 **RATATOUILLE WITH MUSHROOMS:** Add 10 ounces sliced mushrooms to the skillet with the eggplant.

VARIATION 2 **RATATOUILLE CHICKEN BOWLS:** While the vegetables cook, pan-fry about 1 pound diced boneless chicken breast over medium heat until cooked through, about 10 minutes. Plate the ratatouille in bowls and top with chicken.

SHRIMP SCAMPI

This dish is a quick and easy one, but it feels special because it's shrimp scampi! Shrimp scampi seems to me like the kind of dish you order when you're out at a restaurant, so being able to throw together a quick and healthy Paleo version is great. I love the combination of zucchini noodles with butter, garlic, shrimp, and a splash of white wine. Don't forget the fresh parsley to brighten the whole thing up and make it just as beautiful as it is delicious. **SERVES 6**

PREP TIME: 10 minutes
COOK TIME: 10 minutes

NF **30**

2 tablespoons grass-fed butter

1 pound large shrimp, peeled and deveined

2 garlic cloves, minced

Juice of 1 lemon

¼ cup dry white wine (omit if strict Paleo)

2 or 3 large zucchini, spiralized

2 to 3 teaspoons fresh parsley, chopped

PER SERVING Calories 152
Fat 5g, Protein 19g, Sodium 223mg,
Total Carbs 6g, Fiber 1g

1. In a large skillet over medium-high heat, melt the butter. Once it starts to bubble, add the shrimp, cooking on one side for 2 minutes (don't stir yet). After the first side has cooked, add the garlic and flip the shrimp, cooking on the other side for another 2 minutes. Add the lemon juice and wine (if using) and give it a stir.

2. Remove the shrimp from the skillet and set aside, leaving the liquid in the pan. Add the zucchini to the skillet and sauté for 3 to 4 minutes, until fork-tender. Add the shrimp back in and toss to combine.

3. Serve hot with chopped parsley on top.

VARIATION 1 SHRIMP SCAMPI WITH BROCCOLI: To add even more vegetables to this dish, add ½ cup chopped broccoli after you cook the shrimp. You'll probably want to add the juice of another ½ lemon.

VARIATION 2 SHRIMP SCAMPI WITH TOMATOES: Add 1 (14.5-ounce) can diced tomatoes after you've cooked the shrimp on one side.

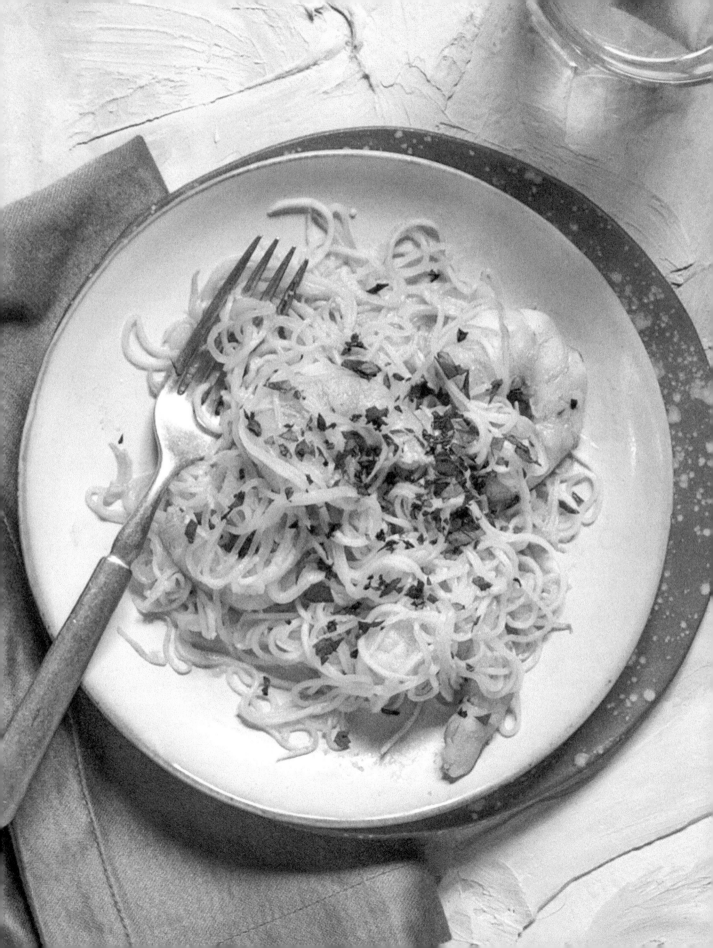

SHORT RIB SUMMER SQUASH NOODLES

Braised short ribs aren't a usual pasta accompaniment, but once I started to think about it, it did make sense—especially if you're using zucchini or summer squash noodles instead of traditional pasta. The beef broth and red wine combine to make a delicious sauce, and the meat from the ribs is incredibly tender. It's a meal so comforting that you might just forget that it's healthy, too. **SERVES 4**

PREP TIME: 10 minutes
COOK TIME: 2 hours, 20 minutes

3 pounds beef short ribs

Salt

Freshly ground black pepper

¼ cup extra-virgin olive oil

1 medium yellow onion, diced

2 garlic cloves, minced

1 (14.5-ounce) can crushed tomatoes (no sugar added)

½ to ¾ cup red wine (omit if strict Paleo)

1½ cups beef broth

3 or 4 summer squash, spiralized

Fresh parsley, chopped, for garnish

PER SERVING Calories 942
Fat 44g, Protein 105g, Sodium 1,001mg, Total Carbs 19g, Fiber 6g

1. Preheat the oven to 350°F.

2. Season the ribs with salt and pepper. In a large Dutch oven over medium-high heat, heat the olive oil. Brown the ribs on each side (this should take 8 to 10 minutes total). Remove the ribs and set aside.

3. Add the onion and garlic and sauté for 3 to 4 minutes, or until the onion is tender. Add the crushed tomatoes and wine (if using). Stir occasionally as you bring the sauce to a simmer.

4. Return the ribs to the pot and cover with the beef broth. Put the lid on the pot and place the whole thing in the oven for about 2 hours, or until the meat falls easily off the bones.

5. Transfer the ribs from the pot to a platter. Put the summer squash in the pot with the sauce and return to the oven to cook for 4 to 5 minutes, or until fork-tender. While the squash cooks, use two forks to shred the meat.

6. Remove the pot from the oven, stir well, and ladle into bowls. Top the summer squash noodles with shredded short ribs, garnish with parsley, and serve.

VARIATION 1 SLOW COOKER SHORT RIBS: Make this meal the night before, or let it cook while you're at work: After you brown the meat, place all of the ingredients except the squash noodles in a slow cooker. Cook on low for at least 8 hours, and then remove the ribs and add the squash noodles to the slow cooker to cook for 5 to 8 minutes, or until fork-tender. Shred the meat and serve as directed in the original recipe.

VARIATION 2 SHORT RIB SUMMER SQUASH NOODLES WITH PEAS: Add 1 cup green peas (thawed if frozen) to the sauce right after you take out the ribs to shred the meat. Stir well and allow to cook for 4 to 5 minutes before adding the noodles.

CINCINNATI CHILI

  Did you know that Cincinnati chili is just chili you put on spaghetti? I had no idea until recently. I make beanless chili all the time, and I love serving it on top of Brussels sprouts or—you guessed it—zucchini noodles. I didn't realize that the whole time I was making Paleo Cincinnati chili. That's one of my favorite things about Paleo food—it's just food, and sometimes you don't even realize you're doing it. **SERVES 4**

PREP TIME: 15 minutes
COOK TIME: 1 hour, 30 minutes

DF **NF**

3 tablespoons extra-virgin olive oil, divided

1 large yellow onion, diced (reserve a couple of tablespoons for topping)

2 garlic cloves, minced

1 pound ground beef, preferably grass-fed

Salt

Freshly ground black pepper

1 (14.5-ounce) can crushed tomatoes (no sugar added)

¼ cup apple cider vinegar

3 tablespoons chili powder

1 tablespoon ground cumin

¼ teaspoon ground cayenne pepper (more or less depending on your heat preference)

1 cup water

2 or 3 large zucchini (or 4 summer squash), spiralized

PER SERVING Calories 405 Fat 19g, Protein 40g, Sodium 1,641mg, Total Carbs 20g, Fiber 8g

1. In a large pot or Dutch oven over medium heat, heat 2 tablespoons of the olive oil and sauté the onion for about 2 minutes, or until tender. Add the garlic and give it another stir.

2. Add the ground beef and allow it to start browning. Season with salt and pepper. Chop it up using a wooden spoon, stirring occasionally. Add the tomatoes and stir to combine. Add the apple cider vinegar, chili powder, cumin, and cayenne pepper. Pour the water in, stir, and bring to a simmer.

3. Allow the chili to cook on medium-low until it begins to reduce and thicken, at least an hour.

4. In a large pan over medium heat, sauté the zucchini noodles with the remaining 1 tablespoon of olive oil for 3 to 4 minutes or until the noodles start to become fork-tender.

5. Serve the chili over the sautéed zucchini noodles, topped with the remaining diced onion.

VARIATION 1 SWEET POTATO CINCINNATI CHILI: While the chili is simmering, spiralize 2 sweet potatoes and toss them in 2 to 3 tablespoons olive oil. Season with salt and pepper and then roast at 450°F for about 15 minutes. Serve in place of the squash noodles.

VARIATION 2 CINCINNATI CHICKEN CHILI: Use ground chicken (or turkey) if you want to lighten up this dish. Follow the steps as written; just substitute 1 pound ground chicken for the ground beef.

BUFFALO CHICKEN ZOODLE BOWL

  This was a weeknight dinner I made on a whim one time, and it soon
became a family favorite. My husband and I are big fans of Buffalo
chicken anything, so I guess it was only a matter of time before I made a
Buffalo chicken zoodle bowl. I like this served right out of the pan, with a
generous drizzle of Paleo Ranch Dressing (page 154). The whole thing is
super quick to whip up, and I hope you enjoy it on a busy weekday night
as much as we do. **SERVES 4**

PREP TIME: 10 minutes
COOK TIME: 15 minutes

1 tablespoon extra-virgin olive oil or ghee

1 pound boneless, skinless chicken breasts or thighs, diced

½ cup grass-fed butter

½ cup Frank's RedHot sauce

3 or 4 large zucchini, spiralized

Salt

Freshly ground black pepper

PER SERVING Calories 483
Fat 35g, Protein 36g, Sodium 1,332mg,
Total Carbs 7g, Fiber 35g

1. In a large skillet over medium heat, heat the olive oil. Add the diced chicken and cook until browned on all sides, about 10 minutes.

2. While the chicken is cooking, in a small pan over medium heat, melt the butter and add the hot sauce to it. Stir well to combine.

3. With a slotted spoon, remove the chicken and set aside. Add the zucchini noodles, cook for 2 to 3 minutes or until the noodles start to become fork-tender, and then stir the chicken back into the pan. Add the butter-hot sauce mixture, season with salt and pepper, and stir gently to combine. Cook for an additional 1 to 2 minutes and serve immediately.

VARIATION 1 CURRY CHICKEN ZOODLE BOWL: Instead of home-made Buffalo sauce, sauté the cooked chicken with 1 minced garlic clove, ¼ cup chicken broth, 1 to 2 teaspoons curry powder, and ¼ cup coconut milk. Add the zucchini noodles, cook as directed, and then serve topped with a sprinkle of crushed red pepper.

VARIATION 2 MEXICAN CHICKEN ZOODLE BOWL: Season the chicken with 2 tablespoons Taco Seasoning (page 155). Cook according to the Buffalo Chicken Zoodle Bowl recipe, omitting the hot sauce and butter. Serve with a squeeze of lime and/or a spoonful of salsa.

TUNA NOODLE CASSEROLE

Tuna noodle casserole is a classic, old-school dish that I feel like everyone should know how to make, except that I didn't know how to make it because my mom never fed it to us. We weren't really noodle casserole people, but I must admit that I always loved the sound of it. Tuna, noodles, cream of mushroom soup, peas—what's not to love? Seriously, those are some of my favorite things. If you did indeed grow up on tuna noodle casserole, then I hope this Paleo version becomes your new tradition. **SERVES 6**

PREP TIME: 15 minutes
COOK TIME: 40 minutes

NF

1 tablespoon grass-fed butter

1 large yellow onion, diced

2 garlic cloves, minced

10 ounces mushrooms, sliced

Salt

Freshly ground black pepper

½ (14.5-ounce) can coconut milk (full-fat)

1 tablespoon arrowroot powder

1 (6- to 8-ounce) can tuna

1 cup green peas (thawed if frozen)

2 eggs, whisked

4 or 5 zucchini, spiralized

PER SERVING Calories 255
Fat 15g, Protein 18g, Sodium 274,
Total Carbs 15g, Fiber 5g

1. Preheat the oven to 400°F.

2. In a large skillet over medium heat, melt the butter and sauté the onion and garlic. After 3 to 4 minutes, add the mushrooms. Season with salt and pepper. Cook for 8 to 10 minutes over medium-high heat, until the mushrooms are nicely browned. Remove them from the pan and set aside.

3. Add the coconut milk and arrowroot powder to the pan. Reduce the heat to medium-low and stir well to get rid of any arrowroot clumps. Remove from the heat and add the tuna, green peas, mushrooms, and eggs. Add the zucchini noodles, and stir gently to combine everything. Season with salt and pepper.

4. Pour the mixture into a baking dish and bake for 25 minutes. Allow to cool slightly before serving.

VARIATION 1 CHICKEN AND MUSHROOM NOODLE CASSEROLE: Instead of tuna, use 6 to 8 ounces canned chicken and add a diced red bell pepper to the skillet along with the mushrooms. Follow the rest of the directions as written.

VARIATION 2 TUNA NOODLE CASSEROLE WITH BROCCOLI: Sauté 1 cup chopped broccoli for 8 to 10 minutes after you remove the mushrooms from the skillet. Remove the broccoli and follow the rest of the recipe as written, remembering to add the broccoli to the skillet before mixing it all together to pour into the baking dish.

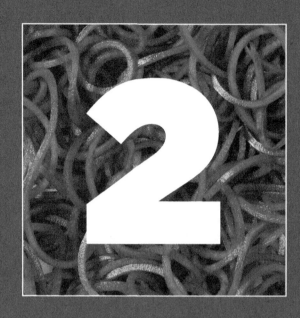

BEETS

Beets can be a little intimidating, because if you aren't prepared to work with them, they can really make a mess. I also think they're one of those vegetables that most people *think* they don't like, until someone else gives them a little push to try them. But they are beautiful and delicious either raw or cooked, which makes them especially great for spiralizing. Most of the raw noodle recipes in this chapter will use blade A (ribbons) or D (spaghetti), because if you're going to eat beets raw, they're just a little better when sliced thin. They have an earthy sweetness that pairs well with a great variety of flavors and textures—from roast beef to fresh herbs and citrus.

Other than their flavor and hearty texture, my favorite thing about beets is their gorgeous color! The red ones (which you'll find most often) are stunning, particularly when cut into lovely noodles. All 10 of these recipes make the most of everything beets have to offer, so if you're a fan, you'll have plenty of inspiration. And if you're not a fan of beets, now you have a reason to try them!

Note: Make sure you peel the beets completely before spiralizing. (This goes for every recipe in this chapter.)

MARINATED BEET NOODLES with GRAPEFRUIT and TARRAGON

 This recipe was inspired by a cocktail I had at Kindred in Davidson, North Carolina—a restaurant that has truly become one of my favorite places in the world. The cocktail was simple, but elegant: grapefruit juice topped with sparkling wine and a sprig of fresh tarragon. The combination of citrus and savory herbs had been on my mind for quite some time, so I couldn't help but incorporate the pairing into a salad. **SERVES 6**

PREP TIME: 10 minutes, plus 15 minutes to marinate

4 beets, peeled and spiralized

1 large grapefruit, segmented

½ cup extra-virgin olive oil

¼ cup rice vinegar

1 tablespoon honey

¼ cup lightly packed fresh tarragon, chopped

Salt

Freshly ground black pepper

PER SERVING Calories 201
Fat 17g, Protein 2g, Sodium 246mg, Total Carbs 12g, Fiber 2g

1. In a large bowl, gently toss the beets and grapefruit to combine.

2. In a smaller bowl, mix the oil, vinegar, honey, and tarragon together. Season with salt and pepper.

3. Pour the vinaigrette over the noodles and grapefruit and toss to combine. Season again with salt and pepper, if necessary. For best flavor, allow to marinate for about 15 minutes before serving.

VARIATION 1 BEET SALAD WITH GRAPEFRUIT AND AVOCADO: Skip the tarragon and serve this salad with a sliced avocado on top.

VARIATION 2 BEET SALAD WITH GRAPEFRUIT AND MINT: If you don't like the flavor of tarragon, use fresh mint instead.

QUICK-PICKLED BEET NOODLES

 I love pickled vegetables so much—carrots, okra, cucumbers (see page 100), onions (see page 156), and beets are definitely up there on my list of favorites. I especially enjoy them as a garnish on a Bloody Mary or almost any other cocktail, but I also love having them as a snack on their own, or as a topping on any number of recipes—lots from *The Big 15 Paleo Cookbook*—but if you want to top your noodle recipes from this book with more noodles, please be my guest! **SERVES 4**

PREP TIME: 10 minutes
COOK TIME: About 30 minutes, plus 1 to 2 hours to chill

DF **NF**

½ cup apple cider or rice vinegar

½ cup water

¼ cup honey

1 knob fresh ginger, peeled and minced

1 tablespoon black peppercorns

1 tablespoon mustard seeds

1 tablespoon ground cumin

Zest of 1 orange

3 beets, peeled and spiralized

PER SERVING Calories 127 Fat 1g, Protein 2g, Sodium 64mg, Total Carbs 28g, Fiber 2g

1. In a small saucepan over high heat, stir gently to combine the vinegar, water, honey, ginger, peppercorns, mustard seeds, cumin, and orange zest. Bring to a boil and remove from the heat.

2. Pack the beet noodles into a clean, dry, heat-proof canning jar (two jars if they don't fit in one). Pour the hot brine over the noodles and allow to cool.

3. Once the jars are at room temperature, cover and chill for 1 to 2 hours.

VARIATION 1 QUICK-PICKLED BEET AND CARROT NOODLES: Instead of 3 beets, spiralize 1 beet and 2 carrots and follow the original recipe instructions.

VARIATION 2 QUICK-PICKLED BEET NOODLE SALAD: Substitute about ½ cup quick-pickled beet noodles for the squash in the Warm Butternut Squash Noodle Salad with Kale and Cranberries (page 76). You can leave the noodles whole or give them a rough chop. I love quick-pickled veggies on top of a kale salad!

CRANBERRY ORANGE BEET SALAD

This salad is an old family favorite. It came from my friend Joan's mother, Margaret, who gave the recipe to my mom years and years ago. My mom calls it "Margaret's Salad." I love dishes like that—the ones that are so familiar and well used that you have to name them after someone you know and love. I added beet noodles to the original recipe to make this one, which I guess you could now call "Megan's Salad." **SERVES 8**

PREP TIME: 10 minutes
COOK TIME: 15 minutes, plus 30 minutes to stand

DF **V**

¾ cup almonds

1 cup plus 3 tablespoons orange juice

6 tablespoons unsweetened dried cranberries

3½ tablespoons extra-virgin olive oil

2 tablespoons vinegar

1 tablespoon grated orange peel

Salt

Freshly ground black pepper

6 cups spinach

3 or 4 beets, peeled and spiralized

3 oranges, peeled and segmented

PER SERVING Calories 184 Fat 11g, Protein 4g, Sodium 204mg, Total Carbs 20g, Fiber 5g

1. Preheat the oven to 350°F.

2. Spread the almonds on a baking sheet in an even layer and toast in the oven until nicely browned, 7 to 10 minutes, stirring halfway through toasting time to ensure even browning. Check frequently near the end to avoid burning. Set aside.

3. In a small saucepan over medium-low heat, gently stir 1 cup of the orange juice together with the cranberries and bring to a simmer. Remove from the heat, let stand for 30 minutes, and then drain.

4. In a small bowl, mix to combine the oil, vinegar, orange peel, and the remaining 3 tablespoons of orange juice. Add the drained cranberries and season with salt and pepper.

5. In a large serving bowl, toss to combine the spinach, beet noodles, orange slices, and dressing. Top with the toasted almonds and serve.

VARIATION 1 CRANBERRY ORANGE BEET SALAD WITH SALMON: To turn this salad into an entrée, add a 4-ounce piece of salmon to each serving. To prepare the salmon, brush with olive oil, season with salt and pepper, and bake at 450°F for 7 to 10 minutes, or until the meat is mostly opaque and flakes easily with a fork.

VARIATION 2 CRANBERRY ORANGE BEET SALAD WITH MASSAGED KALE, CRANBERRIES, AND CARROTS: Add 3 or 4 shaved carrots to the salad for an extra pop of veggies and color. Replace the spinach with 6 cups curly kale. To massage kale, drizzle 1 to 2 tablespoons olive oil over raw kale, massage with your hands for about 5 minutes, and proceed with the recipe as written.

ROASTED BALSAMIC BEET NOODLES

 This is one of the simplest beet recipes you'll find in this book, and it's as delicious as it is easy—all you do is toss beet noodles in a balsamic vinaigrette and then roast them until they're nice and tender and just starting to crisp around the edges. **SERVES 6**

PREP TIME: 5 minutes
COOK TIME: 15 minutes

DF NF V 30

4 beets, peeled and spiralized

½ cup extra-virgin olive oil

¼ cup balsamic vinegar

1 tablespoon Dijon mustard

Salt

Freshly ground black pepper

PER SERVING Calories 177
Fat 17g, Protein 1g, Sodium 275mg,
Total Carbs 7g, Fiber 1g

1. Preheat the oven to 425°F.

2. Put the beet noodles in a large bowl. In a smaller bowl, combine the olive oil, balsamic vinegar, Dijon mustard, salt, and pepper. Pour the balsamic vinaigrette over the noodles and toss thoroughly to combine.

3. Transfer the beet noodles to a baking sheet and pour any balsamic vinaigrette still in the bowl over them. Season again with salt and pepper and roast for 10 to 15 minutes, or until beets are slightly browned around the edges.

4. Remove from the oven and allow to cool slightly. Serve warm.

VARIATION 1 ROASTED BALSAMIC BEET NOODLES WITH BACON: Add about 8 ounces diced bacon to the sheet pan and roast with the beets.

VARIATION 2 ROASTED BALSAMIC BEET NOODLE SALAD: Serve these roasted beet noodles over one or two handfuls of arugula. Make extra balsamic vinaigrette if desired.

BEET NOODLE SALAD with CURRY DRESSING and PISTACHIOS

 This recipe is super delicious. I love pistachios and beets together, and the curry dressing gives it a delightful savory quality and a kick of heat (which you can adjust according to your taste preferences). It's good topped with chicken or shrimp (see the variations), but it's just as satisfying on its own—whether you're serving it as a light lunch or a side dish with a main course. **SERVES 6**

PREP TIME: 5 minutes, plus 10 minutes to rest
COOK TIME: 5 minutes

DF **30**

1 tablespoon extra-virgin olive oil

4 beets, peeled and spiralized

½ cup Paleo Mayo (page 154)

Juice of 1 lemon

1 tablespoon curry powder

¼ teaspoon ground cayenne pepper

Salt

Freshly ground black pepper

1 tablespoon vegetable broth or water

½ cup shelled pistachios

PER SERVING Calories 156 Fat 12g, Protein 2g, Sodium 412mg, Total Carbs 13g, Fiber 2g

1. In a large skillet over medium heat, heat the olive oil and sauté the beet noodles for about 5 minutes, or until beet noodles become fork-tender. Remove from the heat and allow to cool slightly.

2. In a small bowl, mix the mayonnaise, lemon juice, curry powder, and cayenne pepper. Season with salt and pepper and add the broth. Allow to rest at least 10 minutes.

3. Transfer the beet noodles to a large bowl and add the curry dressing. Mix well to combine and serve topped with the pistachios.

VARIATION 1 CHICKEN CURRY BEET NOODLE SALAD WITH PISTACHIOS: Serve this noodle dish topped with 1 to 2 pounds diced cooked chicken breast. You may want to make more dressing for the chicken.

VARIATION 2 CURRY BEET NOODLE SALAD WITH SHRIMP: Serve topped with 1 to 2 pounds cooked, peeled shrimp. Again, you might want some extra dressing with the addition of a protein.

CHILI-LIME BEET NOODLES

 I love the combination of chili and lime—it's my go-to flavor mixture when I want to make something a little Thai-inspired but don't necessarily have all the ingredients for a pad thai or Drunken Noodles (see page 26). These beet noodles are quickly sautéed with a little garlic and oil and then tossed with your favorite chili garlic oil and a generous squeeze of fresh lime juice. **SERVES 4**

PREP TIME: 5 minutes
COOK TIME: 10 minutes

1 to 2 tablespoons extra-virgin olive oil

1 red onion, sliced thin

1 garlic clove, sliced

2 or 3 beets, peeled and spiralized

2 tablespoons chili garlic oil or chili garlic sauce

Juice of 1 lime

PER SERVING Calories 170 Fat 14g, Protein 2g, Sodium 59mg, Total Carbs 12g, Fiber 3g

1. In a large skillet over medium-high heat, heat the olive oil and sauté the onion and garlic. After 2 to 3 minutes, add the beet noodles and continue to cook for about 5 minutes more, or until beet noodles become fork-tender.

2. Add the chili garlic oil and lime juice and toss to combine. Cook for another 2 minutes and serve immediately.

VARIATION 1 CHILI-LIME SHRIMP WITH BEET NOODLES: Add about 1 pound shrimp to the skillet after you sauté the garlic and olive oil. Follow the remaining recipe steps as written.

VARIATION 2 CHILI-LIME CUCUMBER AND CARROT NOODLES WITH CRUSHED ALMONDS: Instead of beets, spiralize 1 cucumber and 2 carrots. Sauté the onion and garlic and then stir in the chili garlic oil and lime juice. Allow to cool slightly and then toss the dressing with the raw cucumber and carrots. Add ¼ cup crushed almonds to garnish.

TWO-BEET BORSCHT WITH CRISPY BEET TOPPING

 This is a variation on the borscht recipe you may have seen in my first book, but here we're doubling down on beets and serving the soup with a crispy beet noodle topping. We're also blending the soup this time so it's nice and smooth. I love the way rich beef broth, beets, and lots of herbs and veggies come together for a healthy, comforting bowl. You can always use your own homemade beef broth, but I find that store-bought is just fine, and it makes this recipe a lot more manageable. **SERVES 6**

PREP TIME: 15 minutes
COOK TIME: 45 minutes

8 cups beef broth

3 tablespoons extra-virgin olive oil, divided

1 medium yellow onion, diced

2 garlic cloves, minced

2 carrots, chopped

2 celery stalks, chopped

1 teaspoon dried oregano

Salt

Freshly ground black pepper

2 dried bay leaves

4 beets, peeled, 3 grated and 1 spiralized

¼ cup fresh dill, minced

2 tablespoons red wine vinegar

PER SERVING Calories 165
Fat 9g, Protein 9g, Sodium 1,287mg,
Total Carbs 13g, Fiber 3g

1. In a medium saucepan over medium-high heat, bring the broth to a boil. Reduce the heat to low and simmer.

2. In a larger saucepan over medium heat, heat 2 tablespoons of olive oil and sauté the onion and garlic for about 5 minutes, until tender.

3. Add the carrots, celery, and oregano. Season with salt and pepper and cook on low for 7 to 8 minutes, or until the veggies become fork-tender.

4. Carefully transfer the simmering broth to the pot with the vegetables. Add the bay leaves and continue to simmer for 10 minutes.

5. Add the grated beets to the soup and simmer for an additional 15 minutes.

6. While the soup is cooking, in the saucepan you heated the broth in, over medium-high heat, fry the spiralized beet noodles in the remaining 1 tablespoon of olive oil until they start to get crispy, 6 to 7 minutes. ➤

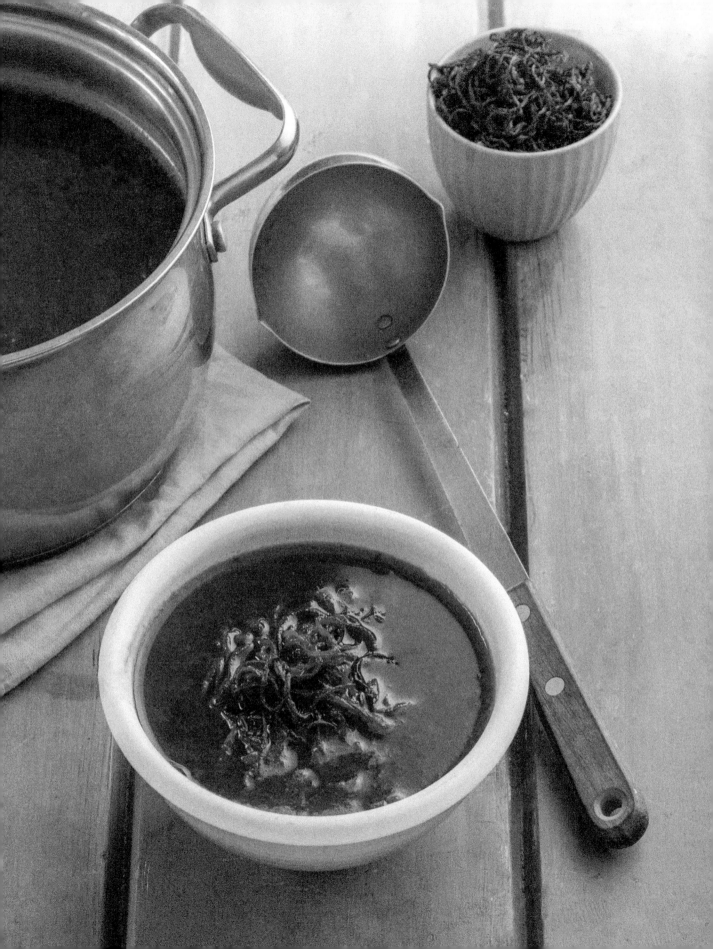

7. Remove the soup from the heat and carefully blend with an immersion blender (you can also transfer it to a blender if you don't have an immersion blender; just be careful and leave enough room that the top doesn't pop off!).

8. Once the blending is complete, add the dill and stir in the red wine vinegar. Serve the soup topped with the crispy beet noodles.

VARIATION 1 **VEGETARIAN BORSCHT:** Make this soup vegan by using veggie broth instead of beef broth.

VARIATION 2 **BORSCHT WITH PAN-SEARED STEAK:** Add 6 ounces sliced, pan-seared steak to each serving.

ROASTED BEET NOODLES with PEAS and FENNEL

 This is the kind of recipe that I want to make in the spring, when you can feel the afternoons warming up but the mornings are still a little chilly. I was in Seattle, on a spring day much like the one I just described, when I fell in love with thinly sliced fennel. My friend Kristan added it to a simple salad, and it was just delicious. The crunchy bite of licorice flavor added an element that was surprising and satisfying. I had to take a page out of her book and add it to these beet noodles roasted with peas. **SERVES 6**

PREP TIME: 10 minutes
COOK TIME: 10 minutes

DF NF V 30

4 beets, peeled and spiralized

1 cup green peas (thawed if frozen)

2 to 3 tablespoons extra-virgin olive oil, plus an extra drizzle for serving

Juice of 1 lemon

Salt

Freshly ground black pepper

1 large fennel bulb

PER SERVING Calories 124 Fat 7g, Protein 3g, Sodium 267mg, Total Carbs 14g, Fiber 4g

1. Preheat the oven to 425°F.

2. In a large bowl, toss the beets and peas in olive oil and lemon juice. Season with salt and pepper. Spread on a baking pan and roast for 5 to 10 minutes, or until beets are slightly browned around the edges.

3. While the noodles are in the oven, slice the fennel bulb very finely—you want to use the white part only. Wash it thoroughly after slicing (dirt can get trapped in the bulb, so I find it easier to wash after I've sliced it).

4. Remove the beets and peas from the oven and return them to the bowl. Toss with the fresh fennel and serve with an extra drizzle of olive oil. Add more salt and/or pepper to taste.

VARIATION 1 BEET NOODLES, PEAS, AND FENNEL WITH BAKED SALMON: Pair each serving of noodles with a 4-ounce piece of salmon. To prepare the salmon, brush it with olive oil, season with salt and pepper, and bake at 450°F for 7 to 10 minutes, or until the meat is mostly opaque and flakes off easily with a fork.

VARIATION 2 BEET NOODLES, PEAS, AND FENNEL WITH GRILLED SHRIMP SKEWERS: Top these noodles with skewers of grilled shrimp: Toss about 1/2 pound large peeled shrimp in olive oil and the juice of 1/2 lemon. Season with salt and pepper, and skewer them onto kabob sticks. Grill for 2 to 3 minutes per side, or until shrimp is pink and opaque.

BEET PASTA WITH LEMON-BUTTER SAUCE

 This beet pasta is a Paleo response to the jealousy I feel anytime I see someone make a gorgeous pasta or gnocchi with beets—it's always this beautiful shade of red, and you know it's just delicious. This recipe uses blade C, so the noodles are a little thicker (like linguini, which is my favorite shape). They're sautéed in butter with lemon and garlic, and they're simple but delightful in flavor—I just love them. **SERVES 4**

PREP TIME: 10 minutes
COOK TIME: 10 minutes

3 tablespoons grass-fed butter

2 garlic cloves, minced

Juice of 2 lemons

3 or 4 beets, peeled and spiralized

Salt

Freshly ground black pepper

PER SERVING Calories 131
Fat 9g, Protein 2g, Sodium 430mg,
Total Carbs 13g, Fiber 3g

1. In a large skillet over medium heat, melt the butter. Sauté the garlic until fragrant, about 1 minute. Add the lemon juice and bring to a low simmer.

2. Add the beet noodles and stir to combine. Sauté for another 5 to 7 minutes or until beet noodles become fork-tender, and season with salt and pepper. Serve immediately.

VARIATION 1 **BEET PASTA WITH WALNUTS AND SAGE:** Sauté the garlic and then add the lemon juice and 2 tablespoons chopped fresh sage. Follow the rest of the original recipe steps. Add ½ cup toasted walnuts as a topping. To toast the walnuts, stir them in a small sauté pan over medium heat until golden and aromatic, about 2 minutes.

VARIATION 2 **BEET PASTA WITH LEMON-BUTTER SAUCE AND CHICKEN:** Add about 1 pound diced boneless chicken breast to the skillet with the butter and garlic. Cook for 8 to 10 minutes, or until the chicken is browned and cooked through. Follow the remaining recipe steps and garnish with a handful of fresh chopped dill.

FLANK STEAK over FRIED BEET NOODLES with HORSERADISH DRESSING

I love flank steak cooked medium-rare with horseradish. I decided to fry beet noodles with some olive oil to take the place of the potatoes that I'd usually serve. The result is a familiar dish with a creative twist—and the horseradish dressing is the perfect way to top it off. This is an impressive special-occasion meal that takes only 30 minutes to throw together. **SERVES 4**

PREP TIME: 15 minutes
COOK TIME: 15 minutes

DF **NF** **30**

1½ pounds flank steak

Salt

Freshly ground black pepper

2 tablespoons extra-virgin olive oil, divided

½ cup Paleo Mayo (page 154)

3 tablespoons horseradish

2 green onions, finely chopped

1 tablespoon red wine vinegar

2 or 3 beets, peeled and spiralized

PER SERVING Calories 546
Fat 31g, Protein 49g, Sodium 689mg,
Total Carbs 16g, Fiber 2g

1. Season the steak with salt and pepper. In a large skillet over medium-high heat, cook the steak with 1 tablespoon of olive oil for 4 to 5 minutes per side, depending on how you like it cooked.

2. While the steak cooks, in a small bowl, mix together the mayonnaise, horseradish, green onions, and red wine vinegar. Season with salt and pepper.

3. Remove the steak from the heat and let rest for about 10 minutes. While the steak is resting, add the remaining tablespoon of olive oil to the skillet and stir-fry the beet noodles for 5 to 7 minutes, or until they begin to crisp.

4. To serve, layer the beet noodles onto plates and top with thinly sliced steak. Spoon the horseradish sauce over the steak or serve on the side.

VARIATION 1 FLANK STEAK OVER FRIED TURNIP NOODLES WITH HORSERADISH DRESSING: Substitute turnip noodles for the beet noodles. Follow the rest of the recipe as written.

VARIATION 2 FLANK STEAK OVER FRIED BEET NOODLES WITH AVOCADO-LIME DRESSING: Instead of horseradish dressing (eliminate the Paleo Mayo, horseradish, green onions, and red wine vinegar), use a food processor or blender to blend 1 avocado, the juice of 2 limes, and some salt and pepper. Serve over the steak.

3
CARROTS

Carrots are one of my favorite vegetables, but unless they're chopped up and used as an aromatic at the beginning of another recipe, I really don't cook with them enough. I usually just eat them raw with a side of Paleo Ranch Dressing (page 154). Oddly enough, they happen to be one of my dog's favorite treats, so we often share a bowl as an afternoon snack (he doesn't eat the dressing, though; he is a dog, after all).

But carrots have a lot to offer as a main ingredient and can be prepared many ways—I particularly enjoy them roasted at a high heat, but you can also pan-fry them, sauté them, bake them in a casserole, and, of course, eat them raw. Carrots are flavorful and delicious, and because they're so good raw, they're easy to use if you're in the mood for something super quick. A couple of my favorites that you'll find in these next few pages: Buffalo Chicken Carrot Noodle Skillet (page 66) and a Carrot Noodle Salad with Tahini-Lime Dressing and Raisins (page 58). Yum! Let's jump in.

Note: When you're planning to spiralize carrots, look for the biggest ones you can find, otherwise your spirals will be more like chips than noodles!

CARROT NOODLE SALAD with TAHINI-LIME DRESSING and RAISINS

 Carrots and raisins go hand in hand. I love the sweetness and texture of both: the crisp, almost juicy crunch of carrots and the chewy dried fruit. This quick carrot noodle salad is dressed with an even quicker dressing of tahini and fresh lime juice. If you haven't used tahini before, it's a loose paste made of sesame seeds, and you can find it in the Asian food section of your local grocery store. **SERVES 4**

PREP TIME: 10 minutes

3 or 4 large carrots, spiralized

1 cup raisins

3 tablespoons tahini

Juice of 2 limes

Salt

Freshly ground black pepper

Fresh cilantro, for garnish (optional)

PER SERVING Calories 215 Fat 6g, Protein 4g, Sodium 358mg, Total Carbs 42g, Fiber 5g

1. In a large bowl, toss the carrots and raisins together.

2. In a smaller bowl, whisk the tahini and lime juice together. Season with salt and pepper. Pour the dressing over the carrot noodles and raisins and toss to combine.

3. Taste and season more if necessary. Garnish with cilantro (if using) and serve immediately.

VARIATION 1 CARROT NOODLE SALAD WITH TAHINI-LIME DRESSING AND AVOCADO: Instead of raisins, toss this salad with 1 diced avocado. Give it an extra squeeze of lime juice and season the avocado with salt and pepper.

VARIATION 2 CARROT NOODLE SALAD WITH TAHINI-LIME DRESSING AND CHICKEN: Up the protein by adding 1 pound diced cooked chicken breast or thighs to the salad. Toss to combine. You may need a little extra dressing to coat the chicken.

CARROT NOODLE SALAD with LEMON VINAIGRETTE

 This salad is a simple but elegant dish that dresses carrot ribbon noodles in a delicious and quick lemon-Dijon vinaigrette. Then everything is tossed together with a couple handfuls of arugula, which is my absolute favorite green—especially when lemon vinaigrette is involved. I like this salad on its own as a snack, but you can easily add virtually any protein to it, including a fried egg, which you'll see in one of the variations below. **SERVES 4**

PREP TIME: 10 minutes

2 tablespoons extra-virgin olive oil

Juice of 1 lemon

1 tablespoon Dijon mustard

Salt

Freshly ground black pepper

3 or 4 large carrots, spiralized

2 cups loosely packed arugula

PER SERVING Calories 94 Fat 7g, Protein 1g, Sodium 380mg, Total Carbs 8g, Fiber 2g

1. In a small bowl, whisk to combine the olive oil, lemon juice, Dijon, and some salt and pepper.

2. In a larger bowl, toss to combine the carrot noodles and arugula. Pour the dressing over the salad and toss again to combine. Season with more salt and pepper, if necessary, and serve.

VARIATION 1 CARROT NOODLE SALAD WITH LEMON VINAIGRETTE AND FRIED EGG: Top each salad with one or two fried eggs. To fry the egg, melt ½ tablespoon grass-fed butter and cook until the egg white has set. Gently flip if you like your eggs over medium; otherwise serve as is (sunny-side up).

VARIATION 2 CHICKEN AND CARROT NOODLE SALAD WITH LEMON VINAIGRETTE: Add 2 (4.5-ounce) cans chicken to this salad. Toss everything together to combine with the dressing.

CARROT NOODLE NESTS

 These carrot noodle nests are an easy way to use up leftover carrots, and you can pair them with almost anything. I like them with chicken or tuna salad or even with a baked egg for breakfast (you can find those recipes in the variations). They're easy to make and a quick way to do something creative with a veggie you probably eat all the time already. **SERVES 6**

PREP TIME: 10 minutes
COOK TIME: 10 minutes

DF NF V 30

3 or 4 large carrots, spiralized

1 tablespoon extra-virgin olive oil

Salt

Freshly ground black pepper

PER SERVING Calories 37 Fat 2g, Protein <1g, Sodium 222mg, Total Carbs 4g, Fiber 1g

1. Preheat the oven to 400°F.

2. In a large bowl, toss the carrot noodles in the olive oil. Season with salt and pepper.

3. Press a small handful of the carrot noodles into each well of a muffin tin (fill 4 to 6 wells). Bake for 8 to 10 minutes, or until the noodles are crisp. Remove from the oven and allow to cool slightly before serving.

VARIATION 1 CARROT NOODLE NESTS WITH BAKED EGGS: Crack an egg over each carrot nest and bake for 8 to 10 minutes, or until the egg white is no longer runny.

VARIATION 2 CARROT NOODLE NESTS WITH CHICKEN SALAD: Serve cooled carrot noodle nests with about ¼ cup of your favorite chicken salad for a quick and easy lunch. For a quick chicken salad, mix 1 (12-ounce) can chicken with 2 tablespoons Paleo Mayo (page 154), ¼ medium yellow onion, finely diced, 1 to 2 celery stalks, diced, and salt and pepper to taste.

CINNAMON-HONEY ROASTED CARROT NOODLES

 My mom made roasted carrots with cinnamon and honey one holiday season, and I remember being completely enamored with them—they didn't even seem like carrots anymore! Who knew that this crunchy root vegetable had the potential to be something so sweet and deeply complex when roasted? This is the noodle version of that recipe—they're delicious on their own or on top of salads. **SERVES 4**

PREP TIME: 10 minutes
COOK TIME: 10 minutes

1 tablespoon extra-virgin olive oil

2 teaspoons honey

½ teaspoon ground cinnamon

Salt

Freshly ground black pepper

3 or 4 large carrots, spiralized

PER SERVING Calories 47
Fat 2g, Protein <1g, Sodium 227mg,
Total Carbs 7g, Fiber 1g

1. Preheat the oven to 425°F.

2. In a small bowl, mix to combine the olive oil, honey, and cinnamon. Season with salt and pepper. Spread the carrot noodles out on a baking sheet, pour the oil and honey mixture over them, and toss to combine.

3. Roast the carrot noodles for 5 to 10 minutes, until golden-brown and a little crispy around the edges, and serve.

VARIATION 1 CINNAMON-MAPLE ROASTED CARROT NOODLES: Use maple syrup in place of the honey for a truly seasonal fall dish.

VARIATION 2 SPICE-ROASTED CARROT NOODLES WITH PISTACHIOS: Add ½ teaspoon cumin and a big pinch of ground cayenne pepper to the carrots along with the cinnamon. Garnish with ½ cup chopped pistachios and the zest and juice of ½ lemon before serving.

VIETNAMESE CARROT NOODLE SALAD

 One of my favorite lunches is a Vietnamese rice noodle bowl. It's fresh, it's crunchy, and it's bursting with awesome flavors and textures—I would eat one every day if I could. But because I shouldn't, I created this dish with carrot noodles instead. The original rice bowls usually have julienned carrots, so that seemed like a natural derivation. You could spiralize all of the veggies this recipe calls for, but I like the difference in texture between carrot noodles, diced cucumbers, and sliced red bell pepper. **SERVES 4**

PREP TIME: 10 minutes

1 garlic clove, minced

¼ teaspoon crushed red pepper

1 tablespoon coconut aminos

Juice of ½ lime

1 tablespoon rice vinegar

1 tablespoon sesame oil

3 or 4 large carrots, spiralized

1 red bell pepper, sliced

1 cucumber, diced

2 green onions, finely chopped

Salt

Freshly ground black pepper

1 handful fresh cilantro, for garnish

Lime wedges, for garnish

PER SERVING Calories 88
Fat 4g, Protein 2g, Sodium 341mg,
Total Carbs 14g, Fiber 3g

1. In a small bowl, mix to combine the garlic, crushed red pepper, coconut aminos, lime juice, rice vinegar, and sesame oil.

2. Divide the carrot noodles among 4 bowls and arrange the bell pepper, cucumber, and green onions over the noodles. Drizzle the dressing over the bowls, season with salt and pepper, garnish each with cilantro and a lime wedge, and serve.

VARIATION 1 **VIETNAMESE CARROT NOODLE SALAD WITH CHICKEN:** Top each serving with 1 sliced boneless chicken breast. To make the chicken: Cook over medium-high heat for 8 to 10 minutes per side in a skillet with olive oil until completely opaque and the juices run clear, and season with salt and pepper.

VARIATION 2 **VIETNAMESE CARROT NOODLE SALAD WITH AVOCADO AND FRIED EGG:** Top each serving with ½ sliced avocado and a fried egg. To fry the egg, melt ½ tablespoon grass-fed butter and cook until the egg white has set. Gently flip if you like your eggs over medium; otherwise serve as is (sunny-side up).

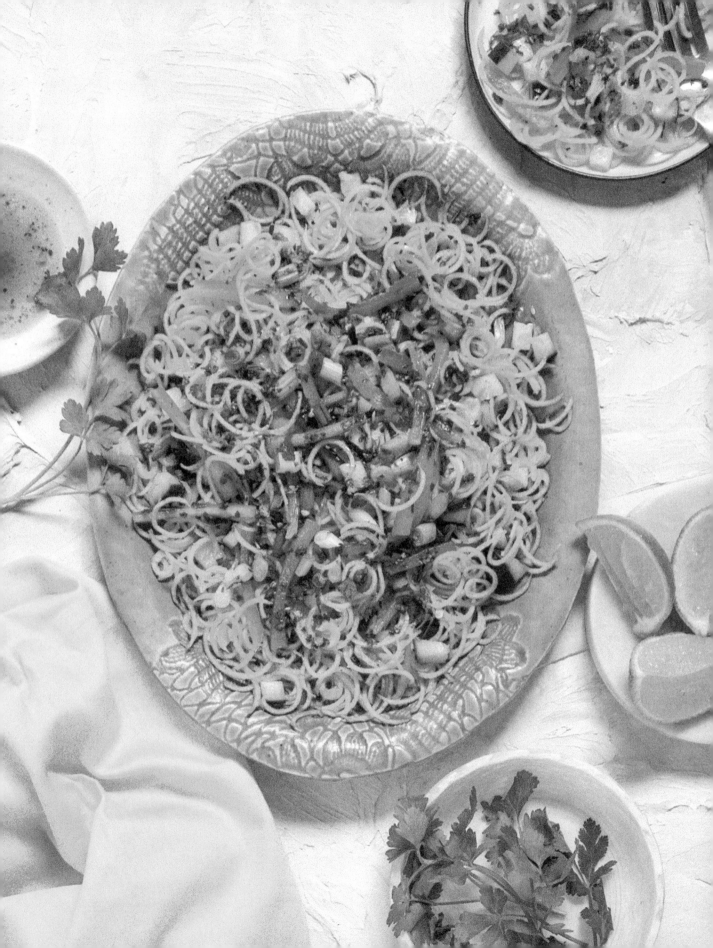

RAINBOW CARROT CURLY FRIES

 Rainbow carrots have got to be one of the prettiest vegetables out there. The purple ones are so crazy looking, and they're even more beautiful when sliced, with their dark purple skin and contrasting orange interiors. This recipe calls for yellow, purple, and orange carrots, which makes for a pretty presentation, but don't worry if you can't find the multicolored ones—regular old orange carrots will do just fine as well. **SERVES 6**

PREP TIME: 10 minutes
COOK TIME: 15 minutes

6 to 8 large rainbow carrots (yellow, purple, and orange), spiralized

¼ cup extra-virgin olive oil

Salt

Freshly ground black pepper

PER SERVING Calories 111 Fat 8g, Protein <1g, Sodium 260mg, Total Carbs 9g, Fiber 2g

1. Preheat the oven to 450°F.

2. In a large bowl, toss the rainbow carrot noodles with the olive oil. Season with salt and pepper.

3. Arrange the carrot noodle curly fries on a baking sheet. Roast for 10 to 15 minutes, or until golden-brown and crisp around the edges, and serve.

VARIATION 1 SEASONED RAINBOW CARROT CURLY FRIES WITH PALEO RANCH: Before baking, toss the carrot noodles with ½ teaspoon each of garlic powder, onion powder, and ground paprika, plus a pinch of ground cayenne pepper. Serve with a side of Paleo Ranch Dressing (page 154).

VARIATION 2 SWEET RAINBOW CARROT CURLY FRIES: Add 2 tablespoons maple syrup and 1½ teaspoons ground cinnamon to the carrots before baking.

CARROT NOODLE EGG DROP SOUP

 Egg drop soup is something that I didn't even think to try to make on my own until very recently. It's so simple: All you do is heat broth (chicken is my favorite) to a simmer, whisk some eggs together, and then gently drizzle the eggs in the broth so they get nice and silky and smooth, not scrambled. It's a great way to use leftover chicken broth, and it adds a little something so it feels a bit more substantial. I've added some carrot noodles to this recipe for even more variation. **SERVES 4**

PREP TIME: 10 minutes
COOK TIME: 5 minutes

DF NF 30

3 cups chicken broth

3 or 4 large carrots, spiralized

2 eggs

Salt

1 green onion, chopped

PER SERVING Calories 86
Fat 3g, Protein 7g, Sodium 936mg,
Total Carbs 7g, Fiber 2g

1. In a medium saucepan over medium-high heat, bring the broth to a boil. Add the carrot noodles and cook for 2 minutes.

2. In a small bowl, whisk the eggs together with a pinch of salt.

3. Remove the broth from the heat and slowly pour the eggs into the soup while stirring gently.

4. Garnish with green onion and serve immediately.

VARIATION 1 **VEGETARIAN EGG DROP SOUP:** Use vegetable broth instead of chicken to make this soup vegetarian.

VARIATION 2 **TRADITIONAL EGG DROP SOUP:** In a saucepan over medium heat, sauté a couple of slices of fresh, peeled ginger and a clove of minced garlic in 1/2 teaspoon olive oil before adding the chicken broth. Omit the carrot noodles, and proceed with the original recipe as written.

BUFFALO CHICKEN CARROT NOODLE SKILLET

If you read my blog or checked out my last book, you know that my husband, Rob, and I are really into Buffalo chicken—so into it, in fact, that we served Buffalo chicken cups at our wedding. Usually we just cook chicken and toss it in some homemade Buffalo sauce, but this dish is new to us, and we love it. Instead of serving the Buffalo chicken with a side of carrots and celery, I spiralized the carrots and fried them up in a skillet, added shredded chicken, and topped it with diced celery and a drizzle of Paleo Ranch Dressing. It's an easy and imaginative way to enjoy a classic. **SERVES 4**

PREP TIME: 10 minutes
COOK TIME: 25 minutes

1 pound boneless, skinless chicken breasts

¼ cup plus 1 tablespoon grass-fed butter

3 or 4 large carrots, spiralized

1 or 2 garlic cloves, minced

¼ cup Frank's RedHot sauce

2 or 3 celery stalks, diced

¼ cup Paleo Ranch Dressing (page 154)

PER SERVING Calories 431
Fat 28g, Protein 34g, Sodium 737mg, Total Carbs 11g, Fiber 3g

1. Steam the chicken breasts by placing them in a steaming basket over a pot of simmering water. Cover and cook for about 15 minutes, or until the juices run clear. Transfer the chicken to a large bowl and allow to cool.

2. In a large skillet over medium heat, melt 1 tablespoon of butter and sauté the carrot noodles. Allow to cook for 3 to 4 minutes, or until carrots are slightly softened. Add the garlic and sauté for 1 minute more.

3. While the carrot noodles are cooking, shred the chicken with two forks.

4. In a separate microwave-safe bowl, melt the remaining ¼ cup of butter by microwaving it for 30 seconds at a time, and then add the hot sauce to it and mix. Pour half of the butter mixture over the carrot noodles and toss to combine. Continue to cook over medium heat.

5. Pour the remaining butter mixture over the shredded chicken and stir well to combine. Add the chicken to the skillet with the carrot noodles, tossing to combine. Continue to stir occasionally for another 3 to 4 minutes, or until the chicken begins to brown and the sauce bubbles a bit. Remove from the heat.

6. Serve topped with the celery and a drizzle of Paleo Ranch Dressing.

VARIATION 1 BUFFALO SHRIMP CARROT NOODLE SKILLET: Instead of steamed, shredded chicken, sauté 1 pound shrimp in the skillet with the carrot noodles and all of the butter mixture. Follow the rest of the original recipe steps as listed.

VARIATION 2 BUFFALO CHICKEN SWEET POTATO NOODLE SKILLET: Substitute 1 large sweet potato (spiralized) for the carrot noodles. (They'll take a little longer to cook, 8 to 10 minutes.)

CHICKEN AND CARROT NOODLE STIR-FRY

 Stir-fry is a good go-to recipe to have when you're busy and need to make a quick but healthy dinner. I love throwing one together with whatever vegetables I have in the fridge—it's a great way to get rid of veggies before they go bad, which is something I'm not always good at. This Paleo stir-fry has all of the flavor and vegetables you're used to, but we're spiralizing the carrots to add a noodle element, and as usual we've replaced the soy sauce with coconut aminos. **SERVES 4**

PREP TIME: 10 minutes
COOK TIME: 20 minutes

2 tablespoons extra-virgin olive oil

1 small yellow onion, sliced

2 garlic cloves, minced

1 small knob fresh ginger, peeled and minced

3 or 4 large carrots, spiralized

1 green bell pepper, sliced

1 head broccoli, cut into florets (save the stem for chapter 7!)

1 (8-ounce) can sliced water chestnuts, drained

1 tablespoon sesame oil

1½ pounds chicken breasts or thighs, diced

½ cup coconut aminos

¼ teaspoon crushed red pepper

Salt

Freshly ground black pepper

PER SERVING Calories 586
Fat 24g, Protein 55g, Sodium 1,276mg,
Total Carbs 38g, Fiber 4g

1. In a large skillet over medium-high heat, heat the olive oil. Add the onion and stir. Cook for 2 to 3 minutes or until the onion is tender, and then add the garlic and ginger. Stir and cook for another minute.

2. Add the carrots, bell pepper, broccoli, and water chestnuts. Cook for about 5 minutes or until the veggies become fork-tender, and remove everything from the skillet.

3. Pour the sesame oil into the skillet and add the chicken. Cook, stirring frequently, until all sides are browned, 8 to 10 minutes.

4. Return the vegetables to the skillet and stir everything together. Add coconut aminos and crushed red pepper, season with salt and pepper, and serve hot.

VARIATION 1 **BEEF AND CARROT NOODLE STIR-FRY:** Instead of chicken, use 1½ pounds thinly sliced steak. (The steak may be done a few minutes sooner than the chicken would be.)

VARIATION 2 **SHRIMP AND CARROT NOODLE STIR-FRY:** Instead of chicken, use 1½ pounds shrimp. (They take only 3 to 4 minutes to cook.)

CARROT PASTA with PEAS and CREAMY GARLIC SAUCE

 What goes better with carrots than peas? This carrot pasta is light and fresh and loaded with—you guessed it—peas! I don't always love coconut cream with savory dishes, but this one has just a tablespoon to make it nice and creamy, which is delicious with the sautéed garlic. And the best part is that carrots take only 2 to 3 minutes to cook, so you could have lunch or dinner ready in no time! **SERVES 4**

PREP TIME: 10 minutes
COOK TIME: 10 minutes

DF NF V 30

3 or 4 large carrots, spiralized

½ cup extra-virgin olive oil

3 garlic cloves, sliced

1 tablespoon coconut cream

1 cup green peas (thawed if frozen)

Salt

Freshly ground black pepper

PER SERVING Calories 291
Fat 27g, Protein 3g, Sodium 336mg,
Total Carbs 12g, Fiber 4g

1. Boil a medium pot of water and add the carrot noodles. Cook for 2 to 3 minutes, or until tender. Drain.

2. In a large skillet over medium heat, heat the olive oil. Add the garlic and stir until fragrant, about 2 minutes. Lower the heat and add the coconut cream. Stir until smooth. Add the peas.

3. Add the drained carrot noodles to the skillet and toss gently to combine. Season with salt and pepper and serve.

VARIATION 1 CARROT PASTA WITH PEAS AND CHICKEN IN CREAMY GARLIC SAUCE: Add about 8 ounces shredded chicken (prepare chicken as in the Buffalo Chicken Carrot Noodle Skillet recipe on page 66) to the skillet with the carrot noodles. Stir to combine and serve hot.

VARIATION 2 CARROT PASTA WITH SHRIMP, PEAS, AND CREAMY LEMON GARLIC SAUCE: Add 1 pound peeled shrimp to the skillet along with the garlic and cook for about 2 minutes per side. Add the zest and juice of 1 lemon to the pan with the coconut milk. Stir well to combine. Follow the remaining recipe steps and serve garnished with a slice of lemon.

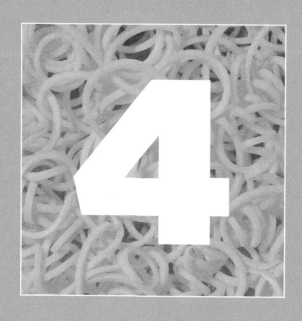

4

BUTTERNUT SQUASH

Butternut squash is not the easiest vegetable to spiralize, but it's one of my favorites. I like how starchy it is compared to zucchini, and I find that the noodles it yields are closer to pasta than any other vegetable, so I love to use it when I'm especially craving noodles.

When you're spiralizing butternut squash, you'll want to follow a few guidelines to get the best results:

1. Choose a medium butternut squash (about 2 pounds) with firm flesh and unblemished skin and peel it thoroughly. Get the skin off, and then peel again to get through the rough exterior. You want to work with only the more vibrant orange flesh—the lighter orange skin (even after you've peeled the first layer) will make it harder to spiralize. So, take the time to peel thoroughly!

2. Next, cut the bulb off the bottom. This is where the seeds are, and the hollow space won't give you enough surface area to spiralize. You can set it aside for other, non-spiralized recipes (and roasted seeds!).

3. Finally, cut the part you're working with in half so you have two pieces that are each a few inches long. This will make it easier to spiralize without losing momentum.

4. Remember that butternut squash noodles take a little longer than zucchini to soften—about 8 minutes.

Now you're ready to cook!

BUTTERNUT SQUASH SALAD with APPLE CIDER VINAIGRETTE

 I love the addition of warm roasted squash or beets to a big salad, so this one is a favorite. You could use any greens you like, but I particularly like the mixture of spinach and arugula. A honey-Dijon apple cider vinaigrette is the perfect complement to the rich butternut squash noodles. This salad is the perfect thing to bring to a holiday potluck or to serve alongside any fall or winter dinner. **SERVES 4**

PREP TIME: 15 minutes
COOK TIME: 10 minutes

1 medium butternut squash, peeled and spiralized (see page 71)

½ cup plus 2 tablespoons extra-virgin olive oil

Salt

Freshly ground black pepper

1 small shallot, minced

¼ cup apple cider vinegar

1 tablespoon Dijon mustard

1 tablespoon honey

1 cup arugula

1 cup spinach

PER SERVING Calories 366 Fat 33g, Protein 2g, Sodium 349mg, Total Carbs 22g, Fiber 3g

1. Preheat the oven to 400°F.

2. In a large bowl, toss the squash noodles with 2 tablespoons of olive oil to coat evenly. Season with salt and pepper and mix again. Transfer to a baking sheet and roast for 8 to 10 minutes, or until squash noodles are fork-tender.

3. While the squash is in the oven, make the vinaigrette. In a small bowl, mix to combine the remaining ½ cup of olive oil with the shallot, apple cider vinegar, Dijon mustard, and honey. Season with salt and pepper.

4. Put the greens in a large bowl, pour some of the dressing over them, and toss to combine. Once the butternut squash is done roasting, remove it from the oven and allow to cool slightly. Add the squash to the salad and toss with the remaining dressing. Serve immediately.

VARIATION 1 SOUTHWESTERN BUTTERNUT SQUASH SALAD WITH HONEY-LIME DIJON AND PEPITAS: Before roasting, toss the squash noodles with 2 teaspoons chili powder. Replace the apple cider vinegar in the dressing with the juice of 2 limes and garnish the salad with ½ cup pepitas (roasted pumpkin seeds).

VARIATION 2 BUTTERNUT SQUASH SALAD WITH APPLE CIDER VINAIGRETTE AND GRILLED CHICKEN: Serve this salad topped with ½ pound grilled chicken breast slices. To grill the chicken, brush with olive oil and season with salt and pepper. Cook on a grill or grill pan over medium heat for 8 to 10 minutes per side, until completely opaque and the juices run clear.

MAPLE-PECAN BUTTERNUT SQUASH CURLS

 These maple-pecan butternut squash curls are really delicious. I'm not always a big fan of maple syrup, but it's so good with roasted squash, especially butternut squash. The end result is kind of like curly fries, but they're practically dessert. You could serve them over a salad or alongside the protein of your choice, but I also really like them on their own as a sweet snack. **SERVES 4**

PREP TIME: 15 minutes
COOK TIME: 10 minutes

1 medium butternut squash, peeled and spiralized (see page 71)

1 to 2 tablespoons extra-virgin olive oil

¼ cup maple syrup

½ cup crushed pecans (toasted or raw)

PER SERVING Calories 271 Fat 16g, Protein 5g, Sodium 8mg, Total Carbs 31g, Fiber 4g

1. Preheat the oven to 400°F.

2. In a large bowl, toss the squash noodles with the olive oil and maple syrup. Transfer to a baking sheet, and bake for 8 to 10 minutes, or until squash noodles are fork-tender.

3. Serve topped with the crushed pecans.

VARIATION 1 BACON-MAPLE-PECAN BUTTERNUT SQUASH CURLS: Add 3 or 4 diced bacon slices to the baking sheet with the squash noodles. Bake for 8 to 10 minutes, or until the bacon is crispy and the squash noodles are fork-tender.

VARIATION 2 HONEY-CINNAMON-PECAN BUTTERNUT SQUASH NOODLES: Instead of maple syrup, use ¼ cup honey and 1 teaspoon ground cinnamon. Bake per the original recipe instructions.

ROASTED MOROCCAN BUTTERNUT SQUASH NOODLES

 The flavor of butternut squash lends itself so well to certain spices—especially cinnamon, ginger, and allspice—so it made sense to whip up a Moroccan spice mix and season some butternut squash noodles with it before quickly roasting them in the oven. These are great both as a snack and as a base for quite a few main dishes (my favorite is the chicken with tomatoes listed in the first variation). **SERVES 4**

PREP TIME: 15 minutes
COOK TIME: 10 minutes

1 medium butternut squash, peeled and spiralized (see page 71)

2 tablespoons extra-virgin olive oil

1 teaspoon ground cumin

1 teaspoon salt

1 teaspoon ground ginger

¾ teaspoon freshly ground black pepper

½ teaspoon ground cayenne pepper

½ teaspoon ground cinnamon

½ teaspoon ground allspice

½ teaspoon ground coriander

¼ teaspoon ground cloves

PER SERVING Calories 130 Fat 7g, Protein 2g, Sodium 589mg, Total Carbs 18g, Fiber 3g

1. Preheat the oven to 400°F.

2. In a large bowl, toss the squash noodles with the olive oil.

3. In a small bowl, mix to combine the cumin, salt, ginger, black pepper, cayenne pepper, cinnamon, allspice, coriander, and cloves. Add the spice mixture to the squash noodles and toss with your hands to combine, ensuring all of the seasoning is evenly distributed.

4. Spread the squash noodles in an even layer on a baking sheet and roast for 8 to 10 minutes, or until the noodles are browned and beginning to crisp.

5. Remove from the oven and allow to cool slightly. Serve warm.

VARIATION 1 MOROCCAN BUTTERNUT SQUASH NOODLES WITH CHICKEN AND TOMATOES: Preheat the oven to 400°F. In a large ovenproof skillet over medium heat, brown 4 chicken thighs in 1 tablespoon ghee, about 5 minutes. Flip them over and add 1 (14.5-ounce) can crushed tomatoes (no sugar added) to the skillet. Reduce the heat to medium-low and add the seasoned butternut squash noodles to the pan. Transfer the skillet to the oven, and cook until the chicken is cooked through, 10 to 15 minutes.

VARIATION 2 ROASTED MOROCCAN BUTTERNUT SQUASH NOODLES WITH POACHED EGGS: If you want turn this into a main course without adding meat, poach eggs to serve on top of the roasted butternut squash noodles. To poach eggs: Bring a large pot of water to a low simmer. Add a splash of white vinegar. Crack one egg into a small dish and use a large spoon to swirl the water into a slow whirlpool. Carefully drop the egg into the water, and without hitting the egg, continue the swirling motion with the spoon. Allow to cook for 1 or 2 minutes, until the whites have set. Carefully scoop the egg out and place it on a paper towel. Repeat with the rest of the eggs you plan to serve.

WARM BUTTERNUT SQUASH NOODLE SALAD
with **KALE** and **CRANBERRIES**

 Kale salads are a new favorite for me—I never thought I liked kale raw, but it turns out if you massage it a bit, it's tender and not at all bitter. I actually like it better raw than cooked, especially when paired with dried cranberries and roasted butternut squash. Traditionally, this salad would be served with diced squash, but I like the addition of squash noodles even more. **SERVES 4**

PREP TIME: 15 minutes
COOK TIME: 10 minutes

1 medium butternut squash, peeled and spiralized (see page 71)

3 tablespoons extra-virgin olive oil, divided

Salt

Freshly ground black pepper

2 cups chopped curly kale

1 cup dried unsweetened cranberries

2 to 3 tablespoons balsamic vinaigrette (see page 47)

PER SERVING Calories 230 Fat 15g, Protein 2g, Sodium 401mg, Total Carbs 23g, Fiber 4g

1. Preheat the oven to 400°F.

2. In a large bowl, toss the butternut squash noodles with 1½ tablespoons of olive oil. Season with salt and pepper, transfer to a baking sheet, and roast for 8 to 10 minutes, or until squash noodles are fork-tender.

3. While the squash is in the oven, in a large bowl, massage the kale with the remaining 1½ tablespoons of olive oil. Use your hands or a wooden spoon to stir continuously for about 5 minutes to soften the leaves. Add the cranberries and roasted squash noodles.

4. Drizzle the balsamic vinaigrette over the salad and toss to combine. Serve immediately, while the squash noodles are still warm.

VARIATION 1 **WARM BUTTERNUT SQUASH NOODLE SALAD WITH KALE, CRANBERRIES, AND CHICKEN:** Serve this salad topped with ½ pound grilled chicken breast slices. To grill the chicken, brush with olive oil and season with salt and pepper. Cook on a grill or grill pan over medium heat for 8 to 10 minutes per side, until completely opaque and the juices run clear.

VARIATION 2 **WARM BUTTERNUT SQUASH NOODLE SALAD WITH STEAK:** Skip the cranberries and serve this salad topped with ½ pound grilled steak. To grill the steak, brush with olive oil and season with salt and pepper. Cook on a grill or grill pan over medium heat for 5 to 7 minutes per side, depending on how you like your steak cooked.

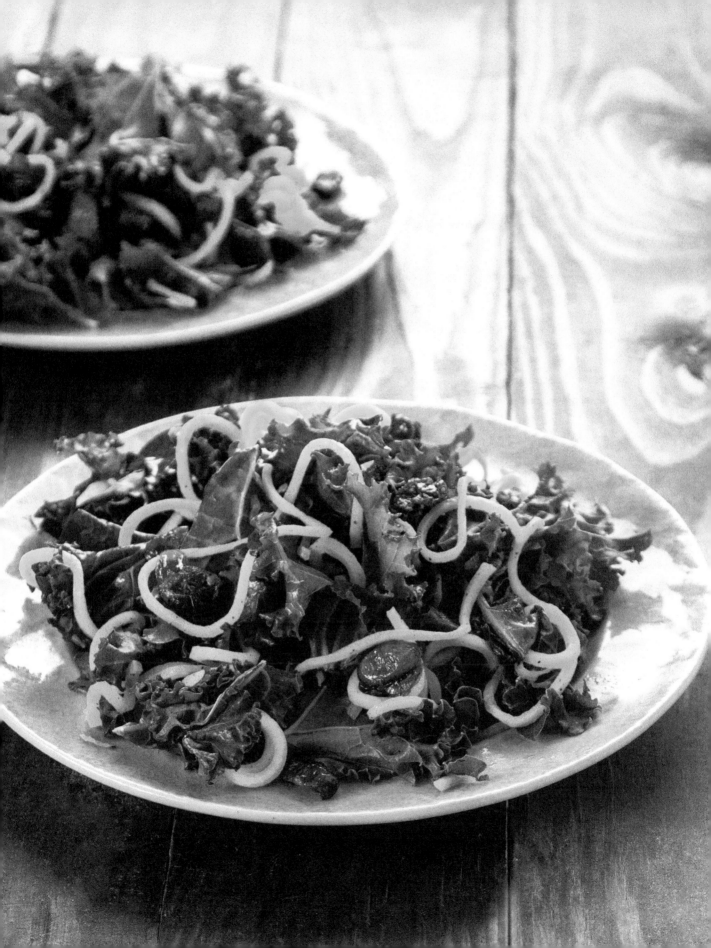

BUTTERNUT SQUASH CURRY NOODLES

   These butternut squash curry noodles are the perfect meal on a chilly day. This dish is easy to customize, so if you like your curry super-hot, you can have it that way, or you can easily keep it on the mild side. Curries are perfect for using up extra veggies you might have hanging around in your fridge. I love this combination of comforting squash noodles, spicy curry sauce, and fresh veggies. **SERVES 4**

PREP TIME: 15 minutes
COOK TIME: 15 minutes

2 tablespoons extra-virgin olive oil

½ red onion, sliced thin

1 tablespoon peeled and minced fresh ginger

2 garlic cloves, minced

1 medium butternut squash, peeled and spiralized (see page 71)

2 tablespoons red curry paste

1 cup canned full-fat coconut milk

1 to 2 tablespoons chili garlic sauce

2 tablespoons fish sauce

2 tablespoons coconut aminos

1 head broccoli, cut into florets and chopped (save the stem for chapter 7!)

2 carrots, sliced

1 red bell pepper, sliced

Fresh lime wedges, for garnish

PER SERVING Calories 347 Fat 24g, Protein 6g, Sodium 1,768mg, Total Carbs 33g, Fiber 7g

1. In a large skillet over medium heat, heat the olive oil and sauté the onion. Cook for 3 to 4 minutes or until the onion is tender, and add the ginger and garlic. Cook for another minute before adding the butternut squash noodles.

2. In a small bowl, mix the curry paste, coconut milk, chili sauce, fish sauce, and coconut aminos. Once the butternut squash noodles have been cooking for about 5 minutes, add the sauce to the skillet. Toss to combine.

3. Add the broccoli, carrots, and bell pepper and give it a good stir. Cook for an additional 3 to 4 minutes, or until the vegetables are brighter in color and fork-tender.

4. Serve hot with fresh lime wedges for squeezing over the bowl.

VARIATION 1 BUTTERNUT SQUASH CURRY NOODLES WITH CHICKEN: Add about 2 pounds diced boneless chicken breast or thighs to the skillet before adding the butternut squash noodles. Cook for 3 to 4 minutes to brown and then add the noodles and continue with the rest of the original recipe.

VARIATION 2 BUTTERNUT SQUASH CURRY NOODLES WITH CABBAGE AND BEAN SPROUTS: Omit the fish sauce for a vegan version of this recipe. Add about 1 cup shredded (or spiralized!) cabbage to the skillet just before serving. Serve with a small handful of bean sprouts (optional; omit if strict Paleo) and the lime wedges, as directed in the original recipe.

BUTTERNUT SQUASH FETTUCCINI
with **MUSHROOMS** and **SAGE**

  This recipe is gorgeous—I just love fresh sage! I think it looks like a cute little lamb's ear, and the light green color and soft texture is lovely, especially when paired with the vibrant orange of butternut squash noodles. I can't get enough sautéed mushrooms. I make them at least once a week and serve them with everything—scrambled eggs, burgers, these squash noodles—and this recipe is one of my favorites. It's especially nice in the fall, but I bet you'll enjoy it all year round. **SERVES 4**

PREP TIME: 15 minutes
COOK TIME: 15 minutes

NF **30**

1 tablespoon extra-virgin olive oil

2 to 3 tablespoons grass-fed butter

12 to 16 ounces mushrooms, sliced

2 or 3 garlic cloves, minced

3 fresh sage leaves, chopped, plus more whole leaves for garnish

Salt

Freshly ground black pepper

1 medium butternut squash, peeled and spiralized (see page 71)

PER SERVING Calories 198 Fat 13g, Protein 5g, Sodium 365mg, Total Carbs 21g, Fiber 4g

1. In a large skillet over medium heat, heat the olive oil and butter. Add the sliced mushrooms and stir. Add the garlic. Stir occasionally as you spread the mushrooms out so they're all making even contact with the skillet. Allow to cook until browned, 6 to 8 minutes.

2. Stir in the sage leaves and season with salt and pepper. Use a slotted spoon to remove the mushroom-sage mixture and set aside. Add the butternut squash noodles to the skillet, and cook for 5 to 7 minutes, or until fork-tender. Season with salt and pepper.

3. Transfer the butternut squash noodles to bowls and top with the mushroom mixture. Garnish each portion with one or two sage leaves and serve.

VARIATION 1 **BACON BUTTERNUT SQUASH NOODLES WITH MUSHROOMS AND SAGE:** Dice 5 or 6 slices of bacon and add to the skillet in place of the olive oil and butter. Sauté the garlic in the bacon fat and add the mushrooms. Stir to combine and then follow the remaining recipe steps as listed in original, adding a little butter or olive oil along with the butternut squash noodles if the pan seems dry.

VARIATION 2 **SAUSAGE BUTTERNUT SQUASH NOODLES WITH MUSHROOMS AND SAGE:** Add about a pound of your favorite sliced, cooked sausage to the skillet a few minutes before serving.

CREAMY PESTO NOODLES

Pesto is one of my favorite sauces to serve with pasta and noodles—it's so easy to make, you don't have to cook it, and it always reminds me so much of my mom, who used to serve pasta with pesto at least once a week when I was growing up. This pesto is made creamier with a couple of avocados and some lemon juice, which keeps it from turning brown and brightens up the flavor. **SERVES 4**

PREP TIME: 15 minutes
COOK TIME: 10 minutes

4 tablespoons extra-virgin olive oil, divided

1 medium butternut squash, peeled and spiralized (see page 71)

2 ripe avocados

1 cup tightly packed fresh basil

2 garlic cloves

3 tablespoons pine nuts

Juice of 1 lemon, or 1 to 2 tablespoons water

Salt

Freshly ground black pepper

PER SERVING Calories 427 Fat 37g, Protein 5g, Sodium 303mg, Total Carbs 28g, Fiber 10g

1. In a large skillet over medium heat, heat 1 tablespoon of the olive oil and sauté the butternut squash noodles. Cook for 5 to 7 minutes, or until fork-tender.

2. In a food processor or blender, process the avocados, basil, garlic, pine nuts, and lemon juice. Keep the food processor running as you drizzle in the remaining 3 tablespoons of olive oil. Season with salt and pepper and add the mixture to the skillet with the butternut squash noodles.

3. Remove from the heat and toss to combine. Serve hot.

VARIATION 1 ROASTED BUTTERNUT SQUASH NOODLES WITH CREAMY PESTO: Instead of sautéing the butternut squash noodles, toss them with 1 tablespoon of olive oil, season with salt and pepper, and roast them on a baking sheet at 415°F for 8 to 10 minutes, or until squash noodles are fork-tender. Toss with pesto and serve.

VARIATION 2 BUTTERNUT SQUASH NOODLES WITH CREAMY CILANTRO-LIME "PESTO": Give this pesto a Latin kick by substituting fresh cilantro for the basil and lime juice for the lemon juice. Omit the pine nuts and serve the noodles tossed in the cilantro-lime avocado sauce and topped with crushed almonds, if desired.

SPICY SAUSAGE SQUASH NOODLES

 This is an easy, one-pot meal that is sure to please everyone in your family. I love spicy Italian sausage, especially when paired with tomato sauce and noodles, so for me this is kind of the perfect weeknight dinner. I also like to serve it when people are visiting, because I think it's such a comforting meal with a clearly home-cooked vibe to it. I hope you get to make this for someone you love soon. **SERVES 4**

PREP TIME: 15 minutes
COOK TIME: 15 minutes

1 to 2 tablespoons extra-virgin olive oil

1 small yellow onion, diced

2 garlic cloves, minced

1 pound hot Italian sausage

1 medium butternut squash, peeled and spiralized (see page 71)

1 (14.5-ounce) can crushed tomatoes (no sugar added)

PER SERVING Calories 562 Fat 39g, Protein 26g, Sodium 1,054mg, Total Carbs 28g, Fiber 7g

1. In a large saucepan over medium heat, heat the olive oil and sauté the onion and garlic for about 5 minutes, until tender. Add the hot Italian sausage to the pot and cook until brown on all sides, 5 to 7 minutes. Remove the sausage from the pot and cut it into slices.

2. Add the butternut squash to the pot and stir to mix with the olive oil, onion, and garlic. Cook for 2 to 3 minutes or until the onion is tender, and add the sausage back in.

3. Add the crushed tomatoes and cook for another 5 minutes or so, or until the sausage is cooked through and the squash noodles are fork-tender. Serve hot.

VARIATION 1 SPICY TOMATO SQUASH NOODLES: Make this dish vegan by skipping the Italian sausage—just make sure to add at least ¼ teaspoon crushed red pepper to make up for the spiciness of the meat.

VARIATION 2 (NOT SPICY) SAUSAGE SQUASH NOODLES: If you aren't into spicy foods, no sweat—just use a mild or sweet Italian sausage.

BROWNED BUTTER(NUT) SQUASH NOODLES
with **FRESH HERBS**

Making browned butter sounds intimidating, but don't worry—it really isn't as tricky as it sounds. Browned butter has a delicious, rich nuttiness that pairs beautifully with butternut squash, especially when accompanied by a bunch of fresh herbs like this recipe calls for. This dish is easy to make but super elegant and full of flavor. It would be perfect for either a quick weeknight dinner or a cozy weekend date night. **SERVES 4**

PREP TIME: 15 minutes
COOK TIME: 10 minutes

NF 30

3 tablespoons grass-fed butter, plus more if needed

1 medium butternut squash, peeled and spiralized (see page 71)

2 tablespoons chopped fresh herbs (a mix of thyme, chives, and parsley)

Salt

Freshly ground black pepper

PER SERVING Calories 182 Fat 9g, Protein 4g, Sodium 264mg, Total Carbs 25g, Fiber 6g

1. In a large skillet over medium heat, brown the butter. Whisk frequently until the butter begins to bubble and foam, 2 to 3 minutes. At this point, some brown milk solids will begin to form at the bottom of the skillet. Remove from the heat and pour the butter into a small bowl.

2. In the same skillet, sauté the butternut squash noodles for 5 to 7 minutes, or until fork-tender, adding a little more butter if the noodles seem dry. Add the browned butter back in and toss to combine. Add the fresh herbs, season with salt and pepper, remove from the heat, and serve warm.

VARIATION 1 BROWNED BUTTER(NUT) SQUASH NOODLES WITH ROSEMARY AND WALNUTS: Add 1 teaspoon chopped fresh rosemary leaves (or ½ teaspoon dried rosemary) to the skillet along with the butternut squash, omitting the herbs from the original recipe. Garnish with 1 cup toasted walnuts. To toast the walnuts: Stir them in a small sauté pan over medium heat until golden and aromatic, about 2 minutes.

VARIATION 2 BUTTERNUT SQUASH NOODLES WITH BROWNED BUTTER–CREAM SAUCE: After removing the browned butter from the heat, add 1 tablespoon canned coconut cream. Stir to combine.

SUN-DRIED TOMATO–BASIL FETTUCCINI

  Sun-dried tomatoes are super easy to find year-round in a jar at your local grocery store. I like adding them to omelets, scrambled eggs, or baked chicken—and they're one of my favorite additions to pasta dishes, which is why I love this butternut squash fettuccini so much. Instead of regular olive oil, you'll cook the squash noodles in the marinated oil from the jar of sun-dried tomatoes, which gives the whole dish a delicious flavor. Then you finish it off with some fresh basil for a quick meal that's as tasty as it is easy! **SERVES 4**

PREP TIME: 15 minutes
COOK TIME: 10 minutes

NF **30**

1 tablespoon grass-fed butter

1 garlic clove, sliced

1 (8-ounce) jar sun-dried tomatoes in oil

1 medium butternut squash, peeled and spiralized (see page 71)

Salt

Freshly ground black pepper

½ cup fresh basil, chopped

PER SERVING Calories 211 Fat 11g, Protein 4g, Sodium 468mg, Total Carbs 30g, Fiber 6g

1. In a large skillet over medium heat, melt the butter. Add the garlic and sauté until fragrant, about 2 minutes, then add the jar of sun-dried tomatoes, including the oil in the jar.

2. Add the squash noodles to the skillet and stir. Season with salt and pepper. Cook for 5 to 7 minutes, or until the noodles are fork-tender.

3. Remove from the heat and add the basil. Toss to combine and serve.

VARIATION 1 SUN-DRIED TOMATO–SAUSAGE BUTTERNUT SQUASH FETTUCCINI: Add about 1 pound of your favorite sliced, cooked sausage to the skillet a few minutes before serving. Garnish with basil as directed in the original recipe.

VARIATION 2 SUN-DRIED TOMATO–BASIL BUTTERNUT SQUASH FETTUCCINI WITH SHRIMP: Add 1 pound shrimp with the sun-dried tomatoes. Season with salt and pepper and cook on each side for about 2 minutes. Remove from the skillet, add the noodles, and cook as directed in the original recipe. Stir in the shrimp and serve warm.

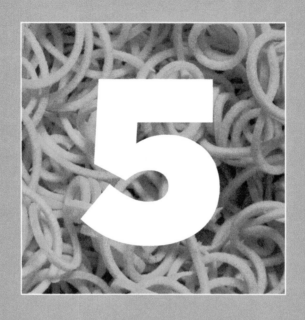

5
SWEET POTATOES

Other than zucchini, sweet potatoes are the main vegetable that comes to mind when I think about spiralizing Paleo food. Sweet potatoes have always been the starch of choice for Paleo eaters, so it only makes sense that we'd be able to come up with 10 delicious sweet potato noodle recipes for you to experiment with!

Sweet potatoes are delicious and easy to prepare, they go well with almost everything, and you can make them sweet or savory—what's not to love? In this chapter, you'll find everything from stews and snacks to "pasta" meal variations, fritters, and even a casserole.

I personally like to peel my sweet potatoes before spiralizing, but it's up to you—the only time I really like having the peel on is if I'm making Sweet Potato Curly Fries (page 88), because I think it gives them great texture and a little extra crunch.

SWEET POTATO HASH BROWN CASSEROLE

 I'm a big fan of casseroles for breakfast, and this one is a variation of one of my favorites from a few years ago. My in-laws always use my recipe when we're together for the holidays, and it's so fun to see something I created turn into a family tradition. I love diced sweet potatoes, but these sweet potato noodles get so much crispier and more flavorful that there's really no substitute for them. **SERVES 4**

PREP TIME: 15 minutes
COOK TIME: 1 hour, 20 minutes

3 tablespoons ghee, divided

¼ medium yellow onion, chopped

1 garlic clove, minced

2 or 3 sweet potatoes, spiralized

1 red bell pepper, diced

Salt

Freshly ground black pepper

8 ounces breakfast sausage (ground sausage, or links with casings removed)

8 eggs

2 tablespoons sliced green onion

PER SERVING Calories 682
Fat 35g, Protein 26g, Sodium 861mg,
Total Carbs 67g, Fiber 10g

1. In a large skillet over medium heat, heat 1 tablespoon of ghee. Sauté the onion and garlic until translucent, about 5 minutes. Add the sweet potato noodles and cook until fork-tender, 7 to 10 minutes. Transfer from the skillet to a baking dish.

2. Add the remaining 2 tablespoons ghee to the skillet and sauté the bell pepper for 2 to 3 minutes. Season with salt and pepper and add to the baking dish as a second layer.

3. Finally, add the sausage to the skillet and cook, stirring often, until no more pink remains, 6 to 8 minutes for ground or 8 to 10 minutes for links. Season with salt and pepper and add to the baking dish as a third layer.

4. Preheat the oven to 350°F.

5. In a medium bowl, whisk the eggs well, season with salt and pepper, and pour over the casserole mixture in the baking dish.

6. Bake for 50 to 70 minutes, or until the eggs are no longer runny. Serve hot, garnished with a sprinkle of sliced green onion.

VARIATION 1 VEGGIE SWEET POTATO HASH BROWN CASSEROLE: For a vegetarian casserole, use 10 ounces sliced mushrooms instead of the sausage.

VARIATION 2 SWEET POTATO AND CARROT NOODLE HASH BROWN CASSEROLE: Use 1 spiralized sweet potato and 2 or 3 spiralized carrots instead of all sweet potatoes. To make this recipe in advance, prepare through step 3 and then cover and refrigerate overnight. Remove the casserole from the refrigerator while the oven preheats, add the eggs, and bake as directed in the original recipe.

SWEET POTATO CURLY FRIES

 Curly fries were always something I thought you had to get in a restaurant or from the frozen food section at the grocery store, but now that I have a spiralizer it's no big deal to whip up a batch of homemade ones! I use blade C because it creates noodles that are closest in size and shape to regular curly fries. After you spiralize them, use scissors or a small knife to cut the noodles into shorter pieces. **SERVES 4**

PREP TIME: 10 minutes
COOK TIME: 10 minutes

3 or 4 sweet potatoes, spiralized and trimmed

2 to 3 tablespoons extra-virgin olive oil

Salt

Freshly ground black pepper

PER SERVING Calories 356 Fat 11g, Protein 3g, Sodium 311mg, Total Carbs 63g, Fiber 9g

1. Preheat the oven to 425°F.

2. In a large bowl, toss to combine the trimmed sweet potato noodles and olive oil. Season with salt and pepper and transfer to a baking sheet.

3. Bake for 10 to 12 minutes, or until the sweet potato curly fries are golden and beginning to crisp. Remove from the oven and allow to cool slightly before serving.

VARIATION 1 **SWEET POTATO CURRY FRIES:** Add 1 tablespoon curry powder and ¼ teaspoon crushed red pepper (if you like it spicier) to the sweet potato fries before baking.

VARIATION 2 **CHILI FRIES:** Serve these sweet potato curly fries with a couple of scoops of chili (page 134—omit the turnips if you wish). Don't forget to grab a fork!

SPIRALIZED SWEET POTATO FRITTERS

 These spiralized sweet potato fritters make an excellent appetizer, side dish, or part of a main course—you can serve them with eggs, chicken, tuna salad, or alongside bunless burgers, to name a few ideas. They're easy to dress up, and with the addition of a little drizzle of Paleo Ranch Dressing (page 154) and a couple of sliced green onions, they're pretty close to perfect. **SERVES 4**

PREP TIME: 10 minutes
COOK TIME: 15 minutes

DF **NF** **30**

1 large sweet potato, spiralized

1 egg, whisked

1 teaspoon garlic powder

1 teaspoon onion powder

Salt

Freshly ground black pepper

1 tablespoon extra-virgin olive oil

PER SERVING Calories 140
Fat 5g, Protein 4g, Sodium 343mg,
Total Carbs 22g, Fiber 3g

1. In a large bowl, toss to combine the sweet potato noodles with the egg, garlic powder, and onion powder and season with salt and pepper.

2. In a large skillet over medium-high heat, heat the olive oil. Create patties about the size of your palm with ¼ cup of the sweet potato noodles and gently place in the hot oil. Cook for 4 to 6 minutes, or until most of the surface is browned and the edges begin to crisp. Carefully flip and cook for another 4 to 6 minutes on the other side. Remove from the skillet and serve hot.

VARIATION 1 **SPIRALIZED SWEET POTATO FRITTER AND EGG SAMMIES:** Serve these sweet potato fritters as an open-faced breakfast sandwich with 2 pieces of cooked bacon, some lettuce, a slice of tomato, and a fried egg on top. To fry an egg, crack it right into the pan with a little grass-fed butter and cook on one side until the white is no longer runny. Carefully flip and cook for 1 to 2 minutes on the other side, depending on how done you want the yolk.

VARIATION 2 **SPIRALIZED SWEET POTATO FRITTERS WITH AVOCADO AND TOMATO:** Serve the sweet potato fritters topped with a quick salad of 1 diced avocado, 1 or 2 diced Roma tomatoes, and a drizzle of balsamic vinaigrette (see page 47). Top with chopped basil as a garnish.

BEEF STEW with SWEET POTATO NOODLES

I make this stew at least once a week during the winter, and I love the addition of sweet potato noodles. They give it an extra level of heartiness that is so delicious and keep this a one-pot recipe. This is the perfect Sunday night dinner—I make a big batch and have the leftovers for lunch the rest of the week! **SERVES 4**

PREP TIME: 10 minutes
COOK TIME: 30 minutes

DF **NF**

2 to 3 tablespoons extra-virgin olive oil

1 medium yellow onion, diced

2 or 3 garlic cloves

2 or 3 sweet potatoes, spiralized

1 pound beef stew meat

1 (28-ounce) can crushed or diced tomatoes (no sugar added)

1 tablespoon chili powder

½ tablespoon ground cumin

Salt

Freshly ground black pepper

1 to 2 cups beef broth

½ cup green peas (thawed if frozen)

PER SERVING Calories 570 Fat 20g, Protein 43g, Sodium 793mg, Total Carbs 57g, Fiber 11g

1. In a large pot over medium heat, heat the olive oil and sauté the onion and garlic together, until translucent, for about 5 minutes. Add the sweet potato noodles, sauté for 3 to 4 minutes, or until the noodles start to become fork-tender, and remove the sweet potato noodles, onion, and garlic from the pot and set aside.

2. Add the beef to the pot and allow to brown on all sides. Add the tomatoes, and give everything a good stir. Season with chili powder, cumin, salt, and pepper. Add 1 cup of beef broth, bring everything to a boil, and then reduce the heat to low. Add the peas and simmer for 5 to 10 minutes.

3. Add the sweet potato noodles, onions, and garlic, and continue to simmer for about 10 minutes more. Stir in the remaining cup of beef broth before serving if the stew seems too thick or dry.

VARIATION 1 WHITE CHICKEN CHILI WITH SWEET POTATO NOODLES: Instead of beef stew meat, make this dish with a pound of ground chicken.

VARIATION 2 TRADITIONAL BEEF STEW WITH CARROT NOODLES: Replace the chili powder and cumin with 1 teaspoon each dried thyme and ground paprika. Instead of sweet potato noodles, use 3 or 4 large, spiralized carrots. Add them in 3 to 4 minutes before you're ready to serve. Garnish with a handful of chopped fresh dill.

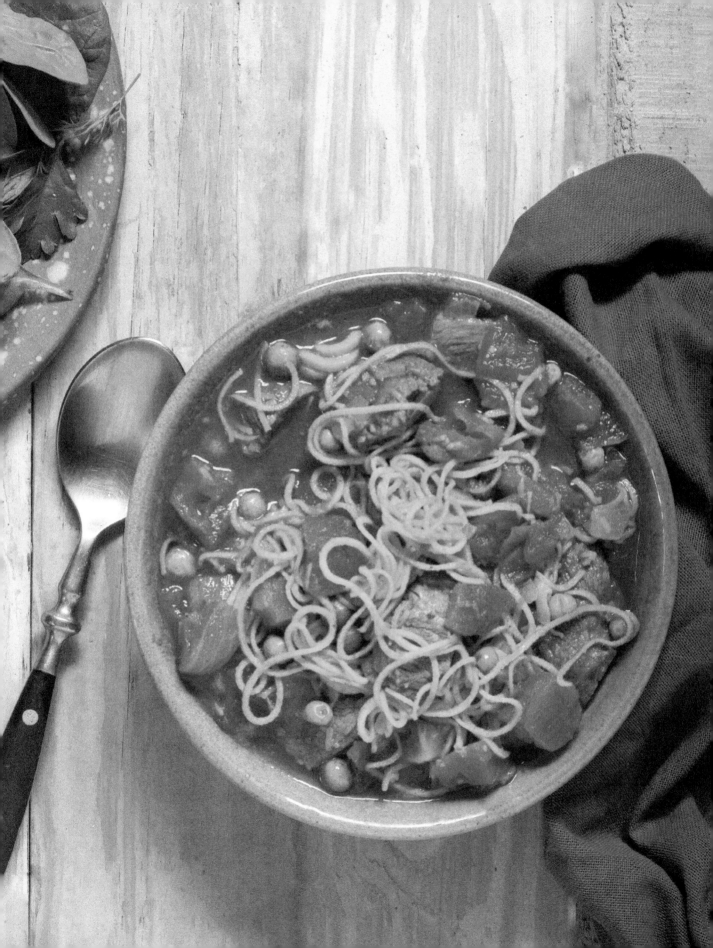

THAI ALMOND SWEET POTATO NOODLE BOWLS

 BLADE I don't use the fettuccini blade on the spiralizer often, but whenever I do I'm always reminded how much I love that shape of noodle, especially with Asian flavors—I think it does such a great job mimicking the shape and texture of pad thai rice noodles. These Thai almond sweet potato noodles combine all the things I love about Thai cuisine, without any grains or excess carbs. **SERVES 4**

PREP TIME: 10 minutes
COOK TIME: 15 minutes

30

1 tablespoon grass-fed butter or extra-virgin olive oil

¼ red onion, sliced thin

1 garlic clove, minced

1 to 2 tablespoons almond butter

Juice of 2 limes

2 tablespoons coconut aminos

½ tablespoon fish sauce

2 or 3 sweet potatoes, spiralized

1 cup bean sprouts (optional; omit if strict Paleo)

3 or 4 green onions, finely chopped

¾ cup sliced almonds

1 lime, quartered

PER SERVING Calories 436
Fat 17g, Protein 12g, Sodium 809mg,
Total Carbs 66g, Fiber 12g

1. In a large skillet over medium heat, heat the butter. Add the red onion and garlic and stir. Sauté for about 5 minutes, until translucent, and add the almond butter, lime juice, coconut aminos, and fish sauce.

2. Add the sweet potato noodles and cook in the sauce for 4 to 5 minutes, or until the noodles start to become fork-tender. Add the bean sprouts (if using) and green onions and cook for an additional 2 to 3 minutes.

3. Remove from the heat, top with the sliced almonds, and serve with a wedge of lime.

VARIATION 1 THAI CHICKEN SWEET POTATO NOODLE BOWLS: Add about 1 pound steamed, shredded chicken breast to this recipe. Steam the chicken breasts by placing them in a steaming basket over a pot of hot water. Cover and cook for about 15 minutes, or until the juices run clear. Remove from the heat and allow to cool.

VARIATION 2 THAI SHRIMP SWEET POTATO NOODLE BOWLS: Add 1 pound peeled shrimp to the skillet after you've made the sauce, but before you put the noodles in. Cook for 2 to 3 minutes per side, or until shrimp is pink and opaque.

FRIED SWEET POTATO "RICE"

Making rice out of veggie noodles is relatively easy and always worth what sometimes ends up being kind of a mess—I love going to Trader Joe's and buying the pre-"riced" cauliflower and broccoli rice, but it's a lot more expensive than making it yourself. I like spiralizing sweet potatoes and then adding them to the food processor until it's the consistency of rice—voila! Now you can make all your favorite rice dishes out of veggies. **SERVES 2**

PREP TIME: 10 minutes
COOK TIME: 20 minutes

NF **30**

2 tablespoons grass-fed butter, divided

½ yellow onion, diced

1 garlic clove, minced

¼ cup carrots, diced

¼ teaspoon peeled, minced fresh ginger

2 sweet potatoes, spiralized and riced

¼ cup green peas (thawed if frozen)

2 tablespoons coconut aminos

1½ tablespoons sesame oil

¼ teaspoon crushed red pepper

2 eggs

2 tablespoons sesame seeds

PER SERVING Calories 617
Fat 31g, Protein 13g, Sodium 776mg,
Total Carbs 74g, Fiber 12g

1. In a large skillet over medium heat, melt 1 tablespoon of butter. Sauté the onion and garlic until translucent, about 5 minutes, and then add the carrots and ginger. Stir to combine and sauté for another 3 to 4 minutes, or until the veggies become fork-tender.

2. Add the sweet potato rice and stir to combine. Add the remaining 1 tablespoon of butter and the peas and cook everything for 5 to 7 minutes. Add the coconut aminos, sesame oil, and crushed red pepper.

3. Move the vegetables over to one side and crack the eggs into the pan. Stir rapidly to scramble and start incorporating the fried rice into the scrambled eggs.

4. Serve hot, topped with sesame seeds.

VARIATION 1 **PORK FRIED SWEET POTATO "RICE":** Add about 1 pound cooked diced pork to the pan about 5 minutes before serving.

VARIATION 2 **BREAKFAST SWEET POTATO RICE:** Sauté ¼ chopped yellow onion and a minced garlic clove in about 1 tablespoon olive oil. Add the sweet potato rice and cook for about 5 minutes. Make room in the center of the pan for the eggs and scramble as directed in the original recipe. Add 2 strips crumbled bacon and stir to combine.

SWEET POTATO LINGUINI
with **MUSHROOMS** and **SPINACH**

 This sweet potato linguini with mushrooms and spinach is really satisfying and quick to throw together—I love anything with sautéed mushrooms, and whenever I can I like to add a couple of handfuls of fresh spinach to a dish to add some extra greens. Sweet potatoes are a great Paleo pasta alternative, and I think using blade C is the easiest way to re-create the feeling of regular noodles. **SERVES 4**

PREP TIME: 10 minutes
COOK TIME: 20 minutes

2 tablespoons extra-virgin olive oil

½ medium yellow onion, diced

2 garlic cloves, minced

10 ounces mushrooms, sliced

2 or 3 sweet potatoes, spiralized

2 cups fresh spinach

Salt

Freshly ground black pepper

PER SERVING Calories 219 Fat 8g, Protein 5g, Sodium 318mg, Total Carbs 36g, Fiber 6g

1. In a large skillet over medium heat, heat the olive oil and sauté the onion for about 5 minutes, until translucent. Add the garlic and mushrooms and cook over medium-high heat for 6 to 7 minutes, or until the mushrooms are browned and crispy.

2. Add the sweet potato noodles and sauté for another 3 to 4 minutes, or until the noodles start to become fork-tender.

3. Add the spinach and stir gently until wilted. Season with salt and pepper and serve hot.

VARIATION 1 SWEET POTATO LINGUINI WITH MUSHROOMS, SPINACH, AND SAUSAGE: Add a little extra protein to this dish by including 3 or 4 sliced Italian sausages to the skillet with the onions.

VARIATION 2 SWEET POTATO LINGUINI WITH MUSHROOMS AND KALE: Swap the spinach for curly kale. Add the kale to the skillet just before the sweet potato noodles and then follow the rest of the recipe as written.

SPAGHETTI with BUTTER and TARRAGON

 This recipe is delicious and incredibly easy to make—butter and tarragon together is such a decadent combination. You can easily add any protein to this dish if you'd like, but I particularly love to use seafood. This recipe is a good starting point because it's gorgeous on its own, but feel free to experiment with your favorite additions—the varieties below include chopped lobster or tuna, but shrimp would be good, too. **SERVES 2**

PREP TIME: 10 minutes
COOK TIME: 10 minutes

NF 30

3 tablespoons grass-fed butter

1 garlic clove, minced

2 or 3 sweet potatoes, spiralized

1 to 2 tablespoons chopped fresh tarragon

Salt

Freshly ground black pepper

PER SERVING Calories 426 Fat 18g, Protein 4g, Sodium 726mg, Total Carbs 64g, Fiber 9g

1. In a large skillet over medium heat, melt the butter. Add the garlic and sauté for 1 minute. Stir in the sweet potato noodles and mix well. Stir every 2 minutes until the noodles are tender, about 5 minutes.

2. Add the tarragon, season with salt and pepper, and serve hot.

VARIATION 1 SWEET POTATO SPAGHETTI WITH BUTTER, TARRAGON, AND LOBSTER: If you're feeling particularly indulgent, add 1 or 2 chopped lobster tails along with the sweet potato noodles. They cook in just a few minutes. They're done when the meat is opaque and firm with no translucency, but watch carefully—they go from done to overdone quickly.

VARIATION 2 SWEET POTATO SPAGHETTI WITH BUTTER, TARRAGON, AND TUNA: Make these noodles with seafood a bit more budget-friendly by serving with a 4-ounce piece of tuna (fresh, or thawed if frozen). To cook the fish, season with salt and pepper and cook for 3 to 4 minutes per side (or less if you prefer medium-rare or rare tuna).

ONE-POT SPAGHETTI and MEATBALLS

 Paleo spaghetti and meatballs is one of my favorite meals to make, with zucchini noodles and sweet potatoes alike. I'm always frustrated with meatballs in Italian restaurants because they usually contain bread crumbs, but I've found that they're just as good without any fillers—just meat and spices and a little salt and pepper. For this recipe, you could easily make the meatballs ahead of time and then simmer everything together in the tomato sauce. **SERVES 2**

PREP TIME: 10 minutes
COOK TIME: 25 minutes

DF **NF**

1 pound ground beef

½ medium yellow onion, chopped

½ cup plus 1 tablespoon chopped fresh parsley

3 garlic cloves, chopped

1 egg, beaten

½ teaspoon dried basil

½ teaspoon dried oregano

½ teaspoon salt

½ teaspoon freshly ground black pepper

1 to 2 tablespoons extra-virgin olive oil

1 (14.5-ounce) can diced tomatoes

½ to 1 teaspoon crushed red pepper flakes (depending on your heat preference)

2 or 3 sweet potatoes, spiralized

PER SERVING Calories 992 Fat 32g, Protein 79g, Sodium 809mg, Total Carbs 98g, Fiber 17g

1. In a large bowl, mix to combine the beef, onion, ½ cup of parsley, the garlic, egg, basil, oregano, salt, and pepper. Roll the mixture into 2-inch meatballs.

2. In a large skillet over medium heat, heat the olive oil. Carefully add the meatballs to the skillet. Brown the meatballs on all surfaces, about 5 minutes per side.

3. Add the diced tomatoes, red pepper flakes, and sweet potato noodles, cook for 5 to 7 minutes more, or until the noodles start to become fork-tender, and remove from the heat.

4. Garnish with the remaining 1 tablespoon of fresh parsley and serve hot.

VARIATION 1 ZUCCHINI SPAGHETTI WITH MEATBALLS: Use 3 or 4 spiralized zucchini instead of sweet potatoes. Cook for 3 to 4 minutes instead of 5 to 7.

VARIATION 2 SWEET POTATO SPAGHETTI WITH TURKEY MEATBALLS: Use ground turkey instead of beef to lighten this recipe up a bit. The cook time will be the same.

CHICKEN ENCHILADA NOODLE BAKE

BLADE Sometimes I'll get a craving for Mexican food and it feels like only tacos or nachos will satisfy it, but lately I've been making this healthier chicken enchilada sweet potato noodle bake instead. It's a Paleo way to incorporate some of those delicious Mexican flavors without grains, sugar, or cheese. You can switch up the vegetables easily, too—the other night I made this with chopped Brussels sprouts instead of sweet potato noodles, and it was just as good. **SERVES 4**

PREP TIME: 10 minutes
COOK TIME: 30 minutes

NF

1 tablespoon ghee

½ red onion, sliced

Salt

Freshly ground black pepper

1 pound boneless, skinless chicken breasts or thighs

2 tablespoons Taco Seasoning (page 155)

2 limes, divided

2 sweet potatoes, spiralized

1 cup Enchilada Sauce (page 156)

2 to 3 tablespoons chopped fresh cilantro, for garnish

PER SERVING Calories 517 Fat 18g, Protein 40g, Sodium 742mg, Total Carbs 59g, Fiber 19g

1. Preheat the oven to 350°F.

2. In a large, ovenproof skillet over medium heat, heat the ghee and sauté the red onion. Cook for 5 to 6 minutes, until translucent, stirring occasionally to keep the onions from sticking. Season with salt and pepper.

3. Season the chicken breasts with the taco seasoning and place them in the skillet, moving the onions around so the chicken gets contact with the pan. Cook for 4 to 5 minutes on each side, until the chicken is browned. Squeeze 1 lime over the chicken and add the sweet potato noodles. Season again with salt and pepper.

4. Pour the enchilada sauce over everything and transfer the dish to the oven. Bake for about 15 minutes, or until the chicken is cooked through. Serve with lime wedges and a sprinkle of cilantro.

VARIATION 1 **CHICKEN ENCHILADA BROCCOLI BAKE:** Instead of sweet potato noodles, sauté the florets from 1 head of broccoli in the ghee with the onion (save the stem for chapter 7 recipes). Remove the florets and onions, brown the chicken as directed, and then return the broccoli florets to the skillet. Follow the rest of the recipe steps as written.

VARIATION 2 **SLOW COOKER CHICKEN ENCHILADA SWEET POTATO CASSEROLE:** Make this recipe overnight or while you're at work by adding all of the ingredients except for the garnishes to a slow cooker and cooking on low for at least 8 hours. For improved flavor and texture, cook the onions and brown the chicken first.

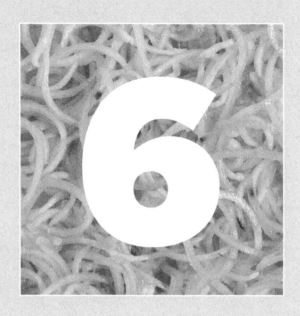

6

CUCUMBERS

Cucumbers are one of my favorite vegetables to spiralize because they're only good raw, which makes these recipes super quick, super light, and super fun to make. They're perfect for when it's too hot outside to even think about cooking, which is how I discovered them in the first place. It was summer in Charlotte, North Carolina, and I ate cucumber noodles nearly every day for lunch.

I don't have a favorite blade to use for cucumber noodles because cook time isn't an issue, so it's just a matter of what kind of noodle you're in the mood for. C provides a nice crunch, but if there's ever a time to use blade A, it's definitely with cucumbers—the wide noodles are so pretty, and I love getting a nice big bowl of ribbon noodles out of just 1 or 2 cucumbers. No matter how you slice them, cucumber noodles will be a fun and fresh addition to your spiralizing repertoire.

QUICK-PICKLED CUCUMBER NOODLES

 Most of my favorite dishes come with pickled cucumbers—I love them on poke bowls and bibimbap—really any Asian dish that's usually served over rice. These quick-pickled cucumber noodles make it easy to enjoy them any time, as a snack or with your favorite meal. **SERVES 4**

PREP TIME: 10 minutes
COOK TIME: 10 minutes, plus 2 hours to chill

DF NF

½ cup red wine vinegar

½ cup water

¼ cup honey

1 to 2 tablespoons salt

1 tablespoon black peppercorns

1 tablespoon mustard seeds

2 large cucumbers, spiralized

PER SERVING Calories 93
Fat <1g, Protein 1g, Sodium 297mg,
Total Carbs 23g, Fiber <1g

1. In a small saucepan, bring the vinegar, water, honey, salt, peppercorns, and mustard seeds to a boil. Turn off the heat.

2. Pack the cucumber noodles into clean jars. Remove the brine from the heat and carefully pour it over the cucumbers. Allow to come to room temperature, cover, and refrigerate for at least 2 hours.

VARIATION 1 QUICK-PICKLED CUCUMBER NOODLES AND RED ONION NOODLES: Add ½ red onion, spiralized, to the jars with the cucumber noodles—use blade A or B to give some texture variation!

VARIATION 2 QUICK-PICKLED OKRA AND CARROTS: Use this brine on whole okra and carrot slices. Try stacking them on toothpicks and serving them with your next batch of Bloody Marys.

CUCUMBER NOODLE SALAD with LEMON and DILL

 I love lemon and dill together—it's such a bright and crisp combination of flavors, and when you pair it with cucumber noodles, it's seriously refreshing. If you can't find fresh dill, a pinch of dried dill would be just fine—just make sure you're using fresh lemon juice! I like squeezing a lemon right over the bowl and seasoning with a pinch of salt and some cracked black pepper. **SERVES 4**

PREP TIME: 10 minutes

2 or 3 large cucumbers, spiralized

Juice of 1 lemon

¼ cup extra-virgin olive oil

2 tablespoons fresh dill, chopped

Salt

Freshly ground black pepper

PER SERVING Calories 149 Fat 13g, Protein 2g, Sodium 301mg, Total Carbs 9g, Fiber 1g

In a large bowl, toss to combine the cucumber noodles with the lemon juice, olive oil, and dill and season with salt and pepper. Serve immediately.

VARIATION 1 CUCUMBER NOODLE SALAD WITH LEMON, DILL, AND TUNA: Serve these cucumber noodles topped with 2 cans of tuna—season with salt and pepper and a small drizzle of olive oil.

VARIATION 2 CHICKEN AND CUCUMBER NOODLE SALAD WITH LEMON AND DILL: Top each bowl of cucumber noodles with about 4 ounces sliced grilled chicken. To grill the chicken, brush with olive oil and season with salt and pepper. Cook on a grill or grill pan over medium heat for 8 to 10 minutes per side, until completely opaque and the juices run clear.

SESAME-VINEGAR CUCUMBER RIBBON SALAD

 I make a variation of this cucumber noodle dish almost every day during the summer—I find that the crunch of raw cucumber is so much more satisfying to me than cooked zucchini noodles, especially when I'm not in the mood to cook. This sesame-vinegar cucumber ribbon salad is tangy and fresh, and using blade A gives you nice wide but thin noodles that are just perfect for twirling with chopsticks. **SERVES 4**

PREP TIME: 10 minutes

DF **NF** **V** **R** **30**

½ cup sesame oil

¼ cup rice vinegar

1 teaspoon chili garlic oil

2 or 3 large cucumbers, spiralized

Salt

Freshly ground black pepper

1 to 2 tablespoons sesame seeds

1 tablespoon chopped fresh cilantro, for garnish

PER SERVING Calories 321 Fat 31g, Protein 2g, Sodium 296mg, Total Carbs 9g, Fiber 2g

1. In a small bowl, stir to combine the sesame oil, rice vinegar, and chili garlic oil.

2. Put the cucumber noodles in a large bowl, pour the dressing over the cucumber noodles, and toss to combine. Season with salt and pepper.

3. Serve the noodles topped with sesame seeds and cilantro.

VARIATION 1 SESAME-VINEGAR CUCUMBER RIBBON SALAD WITH SESAME CHICKEN: Top this salad with diced sesame chicken—dice up about 1 pound boneless chicken breast and sauté in 1 tablespoon olive oil plus 1 tablespoon sesame oil. Cook over medium heat for 7 to 10 minutes, or until all sides of the chicken are browned. Allow to cool slightly before adding to the cucumbers.

VARIATION 2 SESAME-VINEGAR CUCUMBER RIBBON SALAD WITH CHILI-GARLIC SHRIMP: Serve the sesame-vinegar cucumber noodles topped with chili-garlic shrimp—toss 1 pound raw peeled shrimp in 1 to 2 tablespoons chili garlic oil or chili garlic sauce and sauté for 2 to 3 minutes per side, or until shrimp is pink and opaque. Allow to cool slightly before adding to the cucumber noodles.

GAZPACHO with CUCUMBER NOODLES

 I'm a big fan of a nice bowl (or glass, usually) of ice-cold gazpacho in the summer. It's easy to put together, and you don't even have to cook, but you need to chill it for several hours. I like to make this ahead of time so it's ready as soon as I plan to serve it. Instead of adding the cucumber directly to the blender, I kept it out and served it as noodles to give this usually smooth soup a nice crunch. **SERVES 6**

PREP TIME: 15 minutes, plus 4 to 6 hours to chill

1½ pounds tomatoes, chopped

1 small yellow onion, chopped

1 small jalapeño pepper, seeded and minced

1 garlic clove

1 tablespoon sherry vinegar, plus more if needed

Salt

Freshly ground black pepper

¼ cup extra-virgin olive oil, plus more if needed

1 large cucumber, spiralized

PER SERVING Calories 109 Fat 9g, Protein 2g, Sodium 201mg, Total Carbs 8g, Fiber 2g

1. In a blender, purée the tomatoes, onion, jalapeño, and garlic until very smooth, about 2 minutes.

2. With the blender going, add the vinegar and season with salt and pepper. Drizzle the olive oil in as the soup emulsifies to a creamy consistency.

3. Strain the soup and discard the solids. Transfer to a pitcher or bowl and chill for 4 to 6 hours.

4. To serve, fill a bowl with cucumber noodles and pour the gazpacho over it. Season again with salt, pepper, and a splash more vinegar or oil as needed.

VARIATION 1 GAZPACHO WITH CUCUMBER NOODLES AND SHRIMP: Serve this soup topped with 3 or 4 cooked, chilled shrimp and a slice of lemon.

VARIATION 2 SPICY WATERMELON GAZPACHO WITH CUCUMBER NOODLES: Replace half of the tomatoes with watermelon for a fun and fruity twist on this recipe. Add extra jalapeño if you like your food a little spicier.

TOMATO, ONION, and CUCUMBER NOODLE SALAD

 I'm sure you've seen a sliced cucumber and tomato salad with red onion at at least one summer cookout, and this is a spiralized take on that classic. Cucumber noodles are the star of this dish, and if you aren't in the mood to slice the red onion, you could spiralize that too—just make sure to use blade A or D to switch up the texture and size of noodles in the salad. **SERVES 4**

PREP TIME: 10 minutes

2 or 3 cucumbers, spiralized

¼ red onion, sliced thin or spiralized

1 cup cherry tomatoes, halved

½ cup extra-virgin olive oil

¼ cup balsamic vinegar

1 tablespoon Dijon mustard

Salt

Freshly ground black pepper

PER SERVING Calories 266
Fat 26g, Protein 2g, Sodium 343mg,
Total Carbs 11g, Fiber 2g

1. In a large bowl, toss to combine the cucumber noodles, onions, and cherry tomatoes.

2. In a small bowl, mix to combine the olive oil, balsamic vinegar, and Dijon mustard, and season with salt and pepper.

3. Pour the dressing over the salad, toss to combine, and serve immediately.

VARIATION 1 TOMATO, ONION, AND CUCUMBER NOODLE SALAD WITH PALEO RANCH: Instead of balsamic vinaigrette (omit the olive oil, balsamic vinegar, and Dijon mustard), serve this salad tossed with about ¾ cup Paleo Ranch Dressing (page 154).

VARIATION 2 TOMATO, ONION, AND CUCUMBER NOODLE SALAD WITH AVOCADO: Serve this salad with 1 or 2 diced avocados. Sprinkle with a little fresh lime juice to keep the avocado from turning brown.

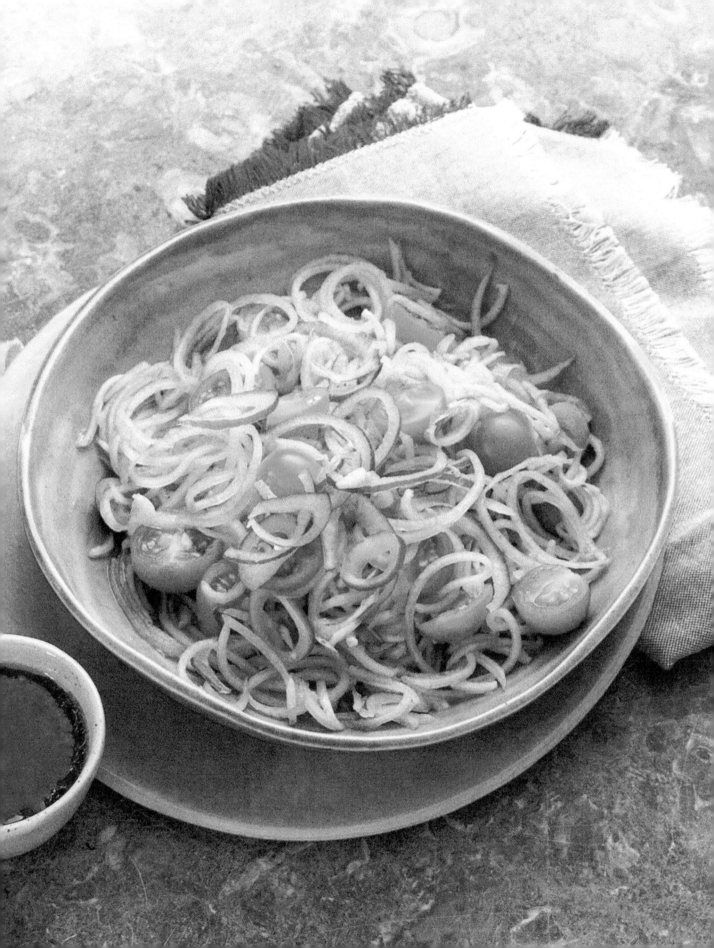

CUCUMBER-MINT GREEN BEAN SALAD

 This salad is full of familiar flavors, but the combination is a bit unusual. I'm a big fan of mixing warm and cool elements, so I love the way the quickly cooked green beans combine with room-temperature or cold cucumber noodles. A hint of fresh mint provides an unexpected pop of flavor that perks up all of the other ingredients. This would be a great dish to bring to your next potluck. **SERVES 4**

PREP TIME: 10 minutes
COOK TIME: 10 minutes

½ pound green beans, cleaned and trimmed

2 large cucumbers, spiralized

1 garlic clove, minced

2 tablespoons extra-virgin olive oil

¼ cup fresh mint, chopped

Salt

Freshly ground black pepper

PER SERVING Calories 104 Fat 7g, Protein 2g, Sodium 299mg, Total Carbs 10g, Fiber 3g

1. In a medium saucepan, quickly blanch the green beans by cooking them in boiling water for about 2 minutes. Drain and then shock them in a bowl of ice water to stop the cooking process.

2. In a large bowl, mix the cucumber noodles and green beans together. Add the garlic, olive oil, and fresh mint. Toss to combine. Season with salt and pepper and serve immediately.

VARIATION 1 CUCUMBER-MINT GREEN BEAN SALAD WITH CHICKEN: Add 4 to 6 ounces canned or shredded chicken to this salad. Toss everything together as directed in the original recipe and serve with a spritz of fresh lemon juice.

VARIATION 2 CUCUMBER-TARRAGON GREEN BEAN SALAD WITH OLIVES: Add ¼ to ½ cup sliced Kalamata or canned olives to this dish and replace the mint with a few tablespoons fresh tarragon.

PORK BÁNH MÌ NOODLES

  My husband always orders a bánh mì sandwich whenever we go to a Vietnamese restaurant, and I'm always jealous—they look so good, but I just can't handle the bread! I used to order a bánh mì burger (pork burger with all the bánh mì fixins) without a bun, so I figured I could easily make a bánh mì sandwich into a Paleo noodle bowl with cucumbers, carrots, and all of the other delicious flavors that make bánh mì so popular. **SERVES 6**

PREP TIME: 10 minutes, plus 2 hours to marinate
COOK TIME: 5 minutes

DF **NF**

2 garlic cloves, sliced thin

¼ cup fish sauce

1 tablespoon honey

4 to 6 green onions, sliced thin

1 tablespoon coconut aminos

1 tablespoon sesame oil

1 tablespoon chili garlic oil or chili garlic sauce, plus more if needed

1½ pounds pork tenderloin, sliced thin

2 or 3 large cucumbers, spiralized

3 or 4 carrots, sliced thin

1 cup loosely packed fresh cilantro, chopped

PER SERVING Calories 265 Fat 9g, Protein 32g, Sodium 1,126mg, Total Carbs 15g, Fiber 2g

1. In a container with a lid, mix the garlic, fish sauce, honey, green onions, coconut aminos, sesame oil, and chili garlic oil. Add the sliced pork and cover. Refrigerate for at least 2 hours.

2. Remove the pork from the refrigerator and cook in a large skillet over medium-high heat until browned on all sides and cooked through, about 5 minutes. Remove from the heat.

3. To assemble the dish, layer the cucumber noodles and sliced carrots into bowls and top with the cooked pork. Add more chili garlic oil or chili garlic sauce if desired, garnish with the cilantro, and serve.

VARIATION 1 PORK BÁNH MÌ NOODLES WITH BEAN SPROUTS AND GINGER: Top these bowls with a handful of bean sprouts (optional; omit if strict Paleo) and about 1 tablespoon pickled ginger from a jar (the kind they serve when you order sushi).

VARIATION 2 PORK BÁNH MÌ NOODLES WITH CHILI-GARLIC AIOLI: Instead of adding more chili garlic oil or chili garlic sauce to this dish on its own, mix 1 to 2 teaspoons with a couple of tablespoons Paleo Mayo (page 154) and serve on the side for dipping.

GARLIC and CHILE-SMASHED CHICKEN with CUCUMBER NOODLES

This is another one of those dishes that you might throw together one time because you have all the ingredients on hand, but before you know it you're writing down the recipe and handing it out to your friends because they want to make it, too. You can adjust the heat of this dish by using more or fewer red chile peppers, but I personally like it really spicy, especially since it's paired with cool cucumber noodles. **SERVES 4**

PREP TIME: 5 minutes, plus 20 minutes to marinate
COOK TIME: 15 minutes, plus 5 minutes to rest

NF

1½ pounds boneless, skinless chicken thighs

1 tablespoon extra-virgin olive oil

3 garlic cloves, smashed and chopped

1 or 2 red chiles, sliced thin (depending on your heat preference)

Salt

Freshly ground black pepper

2 tablespoons ghee

2 or 3 large cucumbers, spiralized

PER SERVING Calories 447 Fat 23g, Protein 51g, Sodium 442mg, Total Carbs 9g, Fiber 1g

1. In a container with a lid, marinate the chicken thighs in the olive oil with the smashed garlic and sliced chiles. Season with salt and pepper. Refrigerate for at least 20 minutes.

2. In a large skillet over medium-high heat, melt the ghee. Add the chicken thighs along with the smashed garlic and chile marinade. Cook for 6 to 7 minutes per side, or until the outside of the chicken is browned and the juices run clear. Remove from the heat, allow to rest for about 5 minutes, and then slice the chicken.

3. In a large bowl, toss the cucumber noodles together with the chicken and some of the chiles and garlic from the pan. Serve while the chicken is still warm.

VARIATION 1 GARLIC AND CHILI-SMASHED SHRIMP WITH CUCUMBER NOODLES: Make this recipe with shrimp instead of chicken. Use 1½ pounds peeled shrimp and marinate it the same way. Cook for 2 to 3 minutes per side, or until shrimp is pink and opaque, and then add the shrimp to the cucumber noodles as directed in the original recipe.

VARIATION 2 GARLIC AND CHILI-SMASHED CHICKEN WITH CARROT NOODLES: Make this recipe with spiralized carrots instead of cucumbers. Use blade C and add the noodles to the skillet with the chicken for 2 to 3 minutes before serving to soften.

CUCUMBER NOODLE SHRIMP COCKTAIL

BLADE

This cucumber noodle shrimp cocktail is more of a salad than a tradi-tional shrimp cocktail. You can serve the cucumber noodles on the side if you want, but I like them either tossed with the shrimp or in a bowl with the shrimp on top. However you prefer to present it, cucumber noodles add a little something to the shrimp and (Paleo) cocktail sauce that we're all so familiar with, and I love turning what is usually an appetizer into a more sub-stantial snack or a light lunch. **SERVES 4**

PREP TIME: 15 minutes

DF **NF** **30**

2 or 3 large cucumbers, spiralized

1 pound cooked shrimp, deveined with the shell off (tails on for easier dipping)

Salt

Freshly ground black pepper

1 lemon, zested and then halved

½ cup tomato sauce (no sugar added)

1 tablespoon horseradish

Hot sauce (depending on your heat preference)

PER SERVING Calories 181 Fat 2g, Protein 28g, Sodium 747mg, Total Carbs 12g, Fiber 2g

1. In a large bowl, season the cucumber noodles and shrimp with salt and pepper and squeeze one of the lemon halves over the bowl. Toss thoroughly.

2. In a small bowl, combine the tomato sauce and the juice of the remaining lemon half with the lemon zest and horseradish. Add hot sauce to taste and season with salt and pepper.

3. Serve the cucumber noodles and shrimp with a dollop of cock-tail sauce, or you can serve the sauce on the side.

VARIATION 1 **CUCUMBER NOODLE SHRIMP COCKTAIL WITH AIOLI:** Make the cocktail sauce into a creamy, indulgent-tasting aioli by mixing 1 to 2 tablespoons Paleo Mayo (page 154) with the tomato sauce, lemon, and horseradish.

VARIATION 2 **CUCUMBER NOODLE GRILLED SHRIMP COCKTAIL:** Grill the shrimp and serve it hot over the cool cucumber noodles. To grill the shrimp, coat in about 1 tablespoon olive oil and place on a grill or grill pan over medium heat for 2 to 3 minutes per side, or until shrimp is pink and opaque (it's a lot easier to skewer them first so they all stay in one place).

CUCUMBER NOODLE POKE BOWL

 Poke bowls are my new favorite thing—I think they're going to be the next avocado toast (which was the next acai bowls, am I right?). When we first moved to California, I probably ate two or three per week, which was delicious, but expensive, and I was consuming way more white rice than I usually do. So now I make them at home, and I substitute cucumber noodles for rice, which saves a lot of carbs and keeps me from spending $15 (seriously—yikes) on a lunch that I can make myself for much, much less. **SERVES 2**

PREP TIME: 15 minutes

2 cucumbers, spiralized

8 ounces sushi-grade ahi tuna, diced

2 or 3 carrots, shredded

1 small daikon radish, shredded

2 tablespoons coconut aminos

1 teaspoon rice vinegar

1 teaspoon sesame oil

½ teaspoon red pepper flakes

2 or 3 green onions, finely chopped

¼ cup seaweed salad (store-bought, optional)

2 to 3 tablespoons pickled ginger (optional)

Sesame seeds, for garnish

PER SERVING Calories 366
Fat 12g, Protein 35g, Sodium 1,035mg,
Total Carbs 31g, Fiber 6g

1. In a large bowl, mix the cucumber noodles with the tuna, carrots, and daikon.

2. In a small bowl, mix the coconut aminos, rice vinegar, sesame oil, red pepper flakes, and green onions.

3. Pour the dressing over the poke bowl ingredients and mix thoroughly. Serve with seaweed salad and ginger (if using) and sesame seeds sprinkled on top.

VARIATION 1 CUCUMBER NOODLE POKE BOWL WITH SALMON: Use raw salmon instead of tuna if you prefer. (Just make sure it's high quality.)

VARIATION 2 CUCUMBER NOODLE POKE BOWL WITH AVOCADO: Dice up an avocado and toss it with the rest of the ingredients and dressing.

CUCUMBER NOODLES IN ALMOND BUTTER SAUCE

 This quick noodle dish is perfect when you're in the mood for something Thai-inspired but want to skip the non-Paleo ingredients so often found in takeout noodle and rice dishes. This dressing is easy to throw together and you can customize it to be spicier if you prefer it that way. **SERVES 2**

PREP TIME: 10 minutes
COOK TIME: 10 minutes

DF **R** **30**

½ cup almond butter

3 tablespoons rice vinegar

1 tablespoon coconut aminos

2 teaspoons sesame oil

¼ teaspoon crushed red pepper (or more depending on your heat preference)

1 lime, halved

2 cucumbers, spiralized

Salt

Freshly ground black pepper

PER SERVING Calories 133, Fat 7g, Protein 4g, Sodium 928mg, Total Carbs 13g, Fiber 2g

1. In a small bowl, mix together the almond butter, rice vinegar, coconut aminos, sesame oil, crushed red pepper, and the juice of one of the lime halves.

2. Place the cucumber noodles in a large bowl and pour the dressing on top. Toss well to combine. Season with salt and pepper and transfer onto plates or bowls for serving. Garnish with a slice of fresh lime.

VARIATION 1 CHICKEN CUCUMBER NOODLES WITH ALMOND BUTTER SAUCE: Serve these noodles with 4 to 6 ounces cubed or shredded cooked chicken. You can make more almond butter sauce if you want, or you can toss everything together in the existing sauce if you prefer.

VARIATION 2 CUCUMBER NOODLES WITH CASHEW BUTTER SAUCE: Use cashew butter instead of almond butter (you can make your own by blending cashews in a food processor) for the sauce. Combine with the noodles as directed in original recipe.

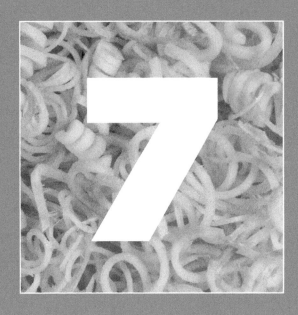

BROCCOLI

If you did a double take when you read that there was a broccoli chapter in a book full of spiralized recipes, you aren't alone. But broccoli noodles are a thing! If you've ever tossed a broccoli stem and wondered if there was anything else you could do with it, then you're in luck—all 10 of these recipes feature noodles made from broccoli stems. I'm a huge fan of saving money and not wasting food, so realizing that the stems of broccoli are not just useable but also delicious was a game changer in my kitchen.

When you're spiralizing broccoli noodles, look for heads of broccoli that are large enough to have a stem that will yield noodles. Pre-chopped broccoli is super convenient, but it's obviously not what you want in this case. Before spiralizing, cut off the florets (but don't throw them away—many of the recipes in this chapter use them in addition to the noodles) and give the stem a quick peel if there are any knobs sticking out. Broccoli noodles need only a few minutes to cook, so before you know it, you'll have a delicious plate full of veggies that you might have otherwise thrown out!

BROCCOLI and ARTICHOKE FRITTATA

  I always keep canned artichoke hearts in my pantry—they make such a nice addition to so many recipes, and they're a great (albeit nontraditional) snack all on their own. Recently, my favorite thing to do with them is add them to a frittata. It reminds me a little of pizza, since I used to love artichokes on my pizza back in my gluten-eating days (and sometimes still, in my gluten-free pizza cheat days). **SERVES 6**

PREP TIME: 10 minutes
COOK TIME: 30 Minutes

DF **NF**

1 to 2 tablespoons extra-virgin olive oil

½ a medium yellow onion

2 garlic cloves, minced

1 head broccoli, cut into florets, stem spiralized

Salt

Freshly ground black pepper

6 eggs

1 (14-ounce) can artichoke hearts

Sliced green onion, for garnish

PER SERVING Calories 186 Fat 11g, Protein 11g, Sodium 400mg, Total Carbs 14g, Fiber 6g

1. Preheat the oven to 350°F.

2. In a cast iron or ovenproof skillet over medium heat, heat the olive oil and sauté the onion and garlic until tender, about 5 minutes. Add the broccoli florets and noodles and stir gently. Season with salt and pepper.

3. In a medium bowl, whisk the eggs.

4. Spread the onion, broccoli, and artichoke hearts evenly in the skillet. Slowly pour the eggs in and increase the heat to medium-high. Season with salt and pepper, and allow to cook until the edges start to pull away from the skillet, 3 to 4 minutes.

5. Transfer the frittata to the oven and cook until the top is no longer runny, 15 to 20 minutes.

6. Allow to cool slightly, garnish with sliced green onion, and serve.

VARIATION 1 BROCCOLI AND ARTICHOKE FRITTATA WITH SAUSAGE: Add ½ pound of your favorite breakfast sausage, crumbled or sliced, to the skillet after the onions, before the broccoli. Cook for 4 to 5 minutes, or until mostly browned. Follow the remaining original recipe steps.

VARIATION 2 BROCCOLI AND ARTICHOKE FRITTATA WITH CHERRY TOMATOES: Sprinkle 1 cup sliced cherry tomatoes on top of the frittata right before you pop it into the oven.

WARM BROCCOLI SALAD with BACON

 Broccoli salad with bacon and a warm vinaigrette is a party staple, so I'm sure you've had something similar at some point. This version feels a little less like a salad because the warm component comes from quickly sautéed broccoli noodles. It's unusual but familiar at once, and I think it might become your new go-to recipe when you're in the mood for a fun and flavorful salad. **SERVES 6**

PREP TIME: 15 minutes
COOK TIME: 10 minutes

DF NF 30

4 to 6 slices bacon, roughly chopped

1 head broccoli, cut into florets, stem spiralized

3 cups spinach

2 carrots, shredded

Salt

Freshly ground black pepper

1 shallot, minced

½ cup extra-virgin olive oil

¼ cup apple cider vinegar

1 to 2 tablespoons honey (depending on your sweetness preference)

PER SERVING Calories 278 Fat 23g, Protein 8g, Sodium 568mg, Total Carbs 13g, Fiber 2g

1. In a large skillet over medium heat, cook the bacon. Add the broccoli noodles after 4 to 5 minutes and cook for another 2 to 3 minutes, or until the noodles are fork-tender and the bacon is crispy.

2. In a large bowl, toss to combine the broccoli florets, spinach, and carrots. Season with salt and pepper.

3. In a small bowl, make the vinaigrette by mixing the minced shallot with the olive oil, apple cider vinegar, and honey. Pour the vinaigrette over the salad.

4. Add the broccoli noodles and bacon, toss to combine, and serve immediately.

VARIATION 1 WARM BROCCOLI SALAD WITH BACON AND CHICKEN: Serve each plate of this salad topped with 4 to 6 ounces sliced cooked chicken (either grilled or steamed).

VARIATION 2 WARM BROCCOLI AND KALE SALAD WITH BACON: Instead of spinach, use 3 cups massaged curly kale. To massage kale, drizzle 1 to 2 tablespoons olive oil over raw kale and massage with your hands for about 5 minutes. Season with salt and pepper.

CREAM of BROCCOLI NOODLE SOUP

 I really love cream of broccoli soup, but I never get it anymore because it is a cream-based soup that usually comes loaded with cheese. It isn't exactly a Paleo-friendly way to enjoy broccoli. I've solved this problem by using coconut milk instead of dairy, and you won't find cheese anywhere in the recipe. To get even more bang for your buck (budget- and nutrition-wise), you'll spiralize the stems and add broccoli noodles to the soup before serving.

SERVES 4

PREP TIME: 10 minutes
COOK TIME: 30 minutes

NF

2 to 3 tablespoons grass-fed butter

1 medium yellow onion, roughly chopped

2 or 3 garlic cloves, roughly chopped

2 heads broccoli, cut into florets, stems spiralized

5 to 6 cups vegetable broth, divided

1 (14.5-ounce) can coconut milk

¼ teaspoon crushed red pepper or ground cayenne pepper (optional)

Salt

Freshly ground black pepper

PER SERVING Calories 432 Fat 36g, Protein 14g, Sodium 1,559mg, Total Carbs 20g, Fiber 7g

1. In a large saucepan over medium heat, melt the butter. Sauté the onion and garlic for about 5 minutes, until translucent. Add the broccoli florets and sauté for another 5 to 6 minutes.

2. Add 5 cups of vegetable broth and the coconut milk. Add the crushed red pepper (if using), season with salt and pepper, and bring to a boil. Reduce the heat to low and simmer for 10 to 15 minutes, or until the broccoli has softened.

3. Use an immersion blender (or a regular blender) to very carefully purée the soup. Add more vegetable broth (or some water) if the soup is too thick for your liking.

4. Add the broccoli noodles and continue to simmer the soup for an additional 4 to 6 minutes. Serve hot.

VARIATION 1 CREAM OF BROCCOLI NOODLE SOUP WITH BEEF BROTH: Make this soup even more flavorful by using beef broth instead of vegetable broth.

VARIATION 2 CREAM OF BROCCOLI NOODLE SOUP WITH BACON: Garnish the soup with a couple of tablespoons of cooked, crumbled bacon. Try cooking the bacon in the oven on a cookie sheet at 400°F for 10 to 15 minutes.

PESTO BROCCOLI SPAGHETTI

   Pesto with broccoli spaghetti is the perfect meal to make when you haven't been shopping in ages and have only random stuff in your fridge and freezer—in my case, that usually means some leftover veggies (like a broccoli stem) and some frozen pesto. You can always make the pesto fresh if you don't have any in your freezer, but don't let that stop you from making a double batch for next time! **SERVES 4**

PREP TIME: 10 minutes
COOK TIME: 10 minutes

DF **V** **30**

½ cup plus 2 tablespoons extra-virgin olive oil

2 heads broccoli, cut into florets, stems spiralized

2 cups fresh basil

¼ cup pine nuts

2 or 3 garlic cloves

2 tablespoons water

Salt

Freshly ground black pepper

PER SERVING Calories 370, Fat 38g, Protein 4g, Sodium 322mg, Total Carbs 8g, Fiber 3g

1. In a large skillet over medium heat, heat 2 tablespoons of olive oil. Add the broccoli florets and cook for 3 to 4 minutes before adding the broccoli noodles. Cook for another 4 to 5 minutes.

2. While the broccoli is cooking, in a blender or food processor, make the pesto by blending the basil, pine nuts, garlic, and water and season with salt and pepper. With the blender running, stream in the remaining ½ cup of olive oil.

3. Remove the broccoli from the heat, add the pesto, and toss to combine. Serve immediately.

VARIATION 1 **PESTO BROCCOLI SPAGHETTI WITH CHICKEN:** Add about 1 pound diced chicken to the skillet with the broccoli florets. Cook until all sides are browned and the chicken is cooked through, 6 to 8 minutes.

VARIATION 2 **WALNUT PESTO BROCCOLI SPAGHETTI:** Use raw walnuts instead of pine nuts when making the pesto.

BROCCOLI BIBIMBAP

(D) BLADE Bibimbap is a Korean rice dish that means "mixed rice," so while this isn't exactly an authentic re-creation, I did my best to capture the flavors in a way that works with the Paleo diet. Broccoli noodles are pulsed in a food processor until they become the consistency of rice and then topped with all the goodness that traditional bibimbap has to offer: garlic, succulent meat, and a fried egg. **SERVES 4**

PREP TIME: 15 minutes
COOK TIME: 30 minutes

2 tablespoons sesame oil

1 tablespoon coconut aminos

1 garlic clove, minced

1 pound ground beef

1 to 2 tablespoons gochujang—Korean chili sauce (depending on your heat preferences)

Salt

Freshly ground black pepper

1 to 2 tablespoons grass-fed butter

4 to 6 ounces shitake mushrooms

2 or 3 carrots, julienned

2 or 3 broccoli stems, spiralized and riced

2 to 4 eggs, depending on how many servings you're making

1 teaspoon rice vinegar

1 tablespoon sesame seeds

PER SERVING Calories 460
Fat 25g, Protein 43g, Sodium 957mg,
Total Carbs 15g, Fiber 4g

1. In a large skillet over medium heat, heat the sesame oil and coconut aminos and sauté the garlic for about 1 minute and then stir in the ground beef. Cook until browned, about 5 minutes, and then add the gochujang. After 5 or 6 minutes, remove everything from the skillet. Season with salt and pepper.

2. Add 1 tablespoon of butter and the mushrooms to the skillet. Cook for 3 to 4 minutes and then use a slotted spoon to remove the mushrooms from the skillet.

3. Add the carrots and sauté over medium-high heat for 2 to 3 minutes, or until the veggies become fork-tender. Use a slotted spoon to remove the carrots from the pan. Add the broccoli rice and sauté for 4 to 5 minutes, or until fork-tender and beginning to brown on some sides. Remove the broccoli rice from the skillet.

4. Fry 1 egg per serving: Crack the eggs right into the pan with a little more butter if necessary, one at a time, and cook on one side until the white is no longer runny. Carefully flip and cook for 1 or 2 minutes on the other side, depending on how done you want the yolk.

5. Assemble the dish by spooning the broccoli rice into bowls and topping with the ground beef, mushrooms, carrots, and egg. Drizzle the rice vinegar over each bowl and garnish with sesame seeds.

VARIATION 1 BIBIMBAP WITH STEAK: Instead of ground beef, use 1 pound thinly sliced steak. Cook until browned and follow the remaining recipe steps.

VARIATION 2 BIBIMBAP WITH SPINACH: Add a couple of handfuls of fresh spinach to the skillet after cooking the carrots. Remove when wilted, after 2 to 3 minutes.

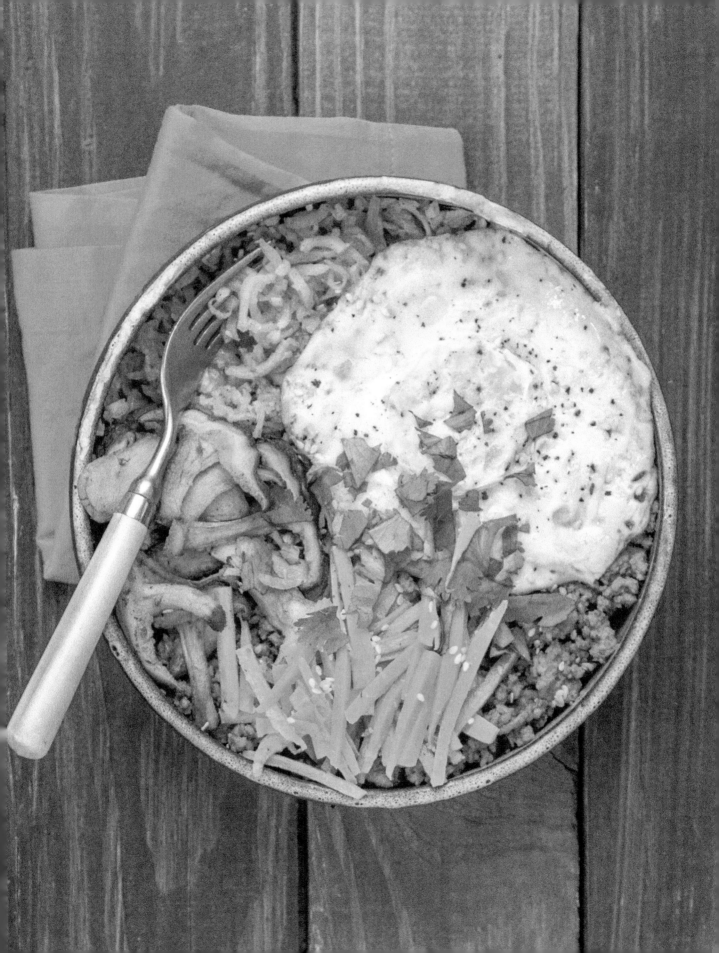

BROCCOLI PASTA WITH LEMON AND KALE

 I've always made kale sautéed with some garlic and a little bit of lemon, but I really love the addition of broccoli noodles and florets—it gives it a nice crunch and makes it feel like more of a main course than a side dish. You can easily add chicken, fish, or any other protein of your choice to make a heartier meal. Either way, broccoli noodles with lemon and kale is a great recipe to make sure you get your greens in (and enjoy them)! **SERVES 4**

PREP TIME: 10 minutes
COOK TIME: 10 minutes

2 tablespoons extra-virgin olive oil

½ medium yellow onion, diced

1 garlic clove, minced

1 head broccoli, cut into florets, stem spiralized

Salt

Freshly ground black pepper

3 to 4 cups curly kale, chopped

Juice of 2 lemons

¼ teaspoon crushed red pepper

PER SERVING Calories 123 Fat 7g, Protein 4g, Sodium 342mg, Total Carbs 12g, Fiber 3g

1. In a large skillet over medium heat, heat the olive oil and sauté the onion and garlic for about 5 minutes, until translucent. Add the broccoli florets and spiralized stems and stir to combine. Season with salt and pepper.

2. Add the kale to the pan and stir until it begins to wilt, about 3 minutes. Add the lemon juice, crushed red pepper, and a bit more salt and pepper if necessary. Cook for 3 to 4 minutes more, or until the kale is wilted and tender. Serve immediately.

VARIATION 1 **BROCCOLI PASTA WITH LEMON AND MASSAGED KALE:** While the broccoli is cooking, pour an additional tablespoon of olive oil over the raw kale. Use your hands to massage the leaves for about 5 minutes, or until the kale turns a brighter shade of green and isn't as rough to the touch. Season with salt and pepper and squeeze lemon juice over the kale leaves. Mix to combine, and serve as a base for the sautéed broccoli.

VARIATION 2 **BROCCOLI PASTA WITH CHICKEN, LEMON, AND KALE:** Add about 1 pound diced boneless chicken thighs or breasts to the skillet after you sauté the onions and garlic. Cook until browned on all sides, add the broccoli florets and spiralized stems, and continue with the recipe as written, until the chicken is cooked through (the chicken should take 6 to 8 minutes total to cook).

BROCCOLI RAMEN BOWL

 This ramen is one of my all-time favorite recipes—I included something similar in my first book and called for zucchini noodles, but I really love the flavor and texture of the broccoli noodles. It takes a little longer to make than most of the recipes in this book, but I think the flavorful broth, tender pork, and variety of toppings are worth the effort. **SERVES 6**

PREP TIME: 15 minutes, plus overnight to chill
COOK TIME: 2 hours

DF **NF**

1 pound pork tenderloin

1 tablespoon salt

2 bunches green onions, (1½ chopped for the broth, ½ sliced for garnish)

1 (2-inch) piece peeled fresh ginger, sliced (about 2 tablespoons)

4 garlic cloves, crushed

7 cups water

3 eggs, for topping

Jalapeño peppers, for topping

Bean sprouts, for topping

Fresh cilantro, for topping

5 tablespoons coconut aminos

2 tablespoons rice vinegar

1½ tablespoons sesame oil

2 or 3 broccoli stems, spiralized (reserve florets for another recipe)

PER SERVING Calories 171 Fat 6g, Protein 22g, Sodium 1,230mg, Total Carbs 6g, Fiber 2g

1. Season the pork with a generous sprinkling of salt and refrigerate overnight.

2. Place the pork in a large saucepan. Add the 1½ bunches green onions to the pot with the ginger, garlic, and water. Bring to a boil, turn the heat down to a simmer, and cook for at least 2 hours (or up to 4 hours).

3. While the broth is simmering, prepare your toppings. Hard-boil the eggs (place in a pot of boiling water and cook for 10 minutes; cool under running water, peel, and halve), slice the jalapeños, and chop the bean sprouts and cilantro.

4. Add the coconut aminos, rice vinegar, and sesame oil to the broth. Continue to simmer and add the broccoli noodles about 5 minutes before you're ready to serve.

5. Remove the pork, slice it, and then transfer it back to the saucepan. Serve the ramen topped with ½ hard-boiled egg per bowl, sliced jalapeño, and chopped bean sprouts and cilantro.

VARIATION 1 **BROCCOLI NOODLE AND FLORET RAMEN:** For an extra boost of veggies, add the florets from the broccoli stem to the broth when you add the coconut aminos, sesame oil, and rice vinegar.

VARIATION 2 **VEGETARIAN BROCCOLI RAMEN BOWL:** Instead of making your own broth, omit the pork and water and use 7 cups vegetable broth. This will save you the overnight marinade step as well, so it's a lot quicker. Follow the rest of the recipe as written, adding broccoli florets and 10 ounces sliced mushrooms to the pot 10 to 15 minutes before serving.

BEEF and BROCCOLI NOODLES

BLADE
Beef and broccoli is one of my favorite dishes to order at a Chinese place, but it's full of cornstarch, soy sauce, and sugar. This beef and broccoli is a simple Paleo stir-fry that incorporates broccoli noodles as well as florets. It's easy to make and is sure to satisfy your Chinese takeout craving without breaking your healthy diet—and you don't even have to pick up the phone! **SERVES 4**

PREP TIME: 10 minutes
COOK TIME: 15 minutes

NF **30**

1 tablespoon grass-fed butter

½ medium yellow onion, diced

2 garlic cloves, minced

1 tablespoon sesame oil

1 pound steak, sliced thin

1 head broccoli, cut into florets, stem spiralized

2 tablespoons coconut aminos

¼ teaspoon crushed red pepper

2 tablespoons sesame seeds, for garnish

2 or 3 green onions, finely chopped, for garnish

PER SERVING Calories 347
Fat 15g, Protein 45g, Sodium 397mg,
Total Carbs 9g, Fiber 3g

1. In a large skillet or wok over medium heat, melt the butter. Add the onion and garlic and sauté for about 5 minutes, until translucent, before adding the sesame oil and steak. Cook for another 5 to 6 minutes, or until the meat begins to brown on all sides.

2. Chop the broccoli florets into bite-size pieces and add them to the skillet. Cook for 3 to 4 minutes and then add the broccoli noodles. Stir to combine and add the coconut aminos and crushed red pepper.

3. Remove from the heat and serve garnished with sesame seeds and green onions.

VARIATION 1 BEEF AND BROCCOLI NOODLES WITH MUSH-ROOMS: Add about 8 ounces sliced mushrooms to the skillet with the broccoli florets in step 2.

VARIATION 2 BEEF AND BROCCOLI NOODLES WITH WATER CHESTNUTS: Add a small can of drained water chestnuts to the skillet a few minutes before serving.

BEEF STROGANOFF

Beef stroganoff is one of those classic recipes that everyone has probably had before, but maybe hasn't made for themselves. This Paleo version is just as delicious and comforting as the original. Instead of egg noodles, we use a spiralized broccoli stem to sneak some vegetables into an otherwise meat- and starch-heavy dish. **SERVES 4**

PREP TIME: 10 minutes
COOK TIME: 30 minutes

NF

4 tablespoons grass-fed butter, divided

1 large yellow onion, sliced thin

2 garlic cloves, minced

1½ pounds beef sirloin steak, sliced

Salt

Freshly ground black pepper

1 cup beef broth

½ cup canned coconut milk

2 large broccoli stems, spiralized

PER SERVING Calories 525 Fat 30g, Protein 55g, Sodium 696mg, Total Carbs 8g, Fiber 3g

1. In a large skillet over medium heat, melt 1 tablespoon of butter. Sauté the onion and garlic for about 5 minutes, until translucent. Add another tablespoon of butter and the steak. Cook until the meat is browned on all sides, about 5 minutes. Season with salt and pepper.

2. Add the broth and coconut milk to the skillet and stir well to combine. Bring to a simmer and cook on low for about 10 minutes, or until the liquid has thickened a bit.

3. While the beef is simmering, bring a small saucepan of water to a boil. Add the broccoli noodles and cook for 2 to 3 minutes, or until tender. Drain and toss with the remaining 2 tablespoons of butter.

4. Transfer the noodles to plates, top with the beef and sauce, and serve.

VARIATION 1 BEEF STROGANOFF WITH MUSHROOMS:
After you cook the onions and garlic, add about 10 ounces sliced mushrooms to the skillet. Cook for 5 to 7 minutes before adding the steak.

VARIATION 2 ONE-POT BEEF STROGANOFF WITH ZUCCHINI NOODLES: Instead of broccoli noodles, serve this over zucchini noodles. Cook them for 2 to 3 minutes, or until the noodles start to become fork-tender, right in the skillet with the beef.

BROCCOLI NOODLE SLAW with ROASTED PORK

BLADE
Pork and slaw are a perfect pairing, and this recipe utilizes broccoli noodles for a little twist. My mom always makes a broccoli slaw for parties, and I included that recipe in my first book, but this one skips the florets and uses the spiralized stems, as well as some julienned carrots and red onion. I like using a dry rub on pork because homemade barbecue sauce can take a long time to make, and it can be hard to find a store-bought sauce without sugar. **SERVES 4**

PREP TIME: 10 minutes
COOK TIME: 50 minutes, plus 10 minutes to rest

DF **NF**

1 pound pork loin

1 tablespoon chili powder

1 tablespoon ground paprika

½ tablespoon garlic powder

½ tablespoon onion powder

½ tablespoon ground cumin

Salt

Freshly ground black pepper

2 tablespoons ghee

1 cup chicken broth

2 large broccoli stems, spiralized

2 or 3 carrots, sliced thin

¼ red onion, sliced thin

½ cup Paleo Mayo (page 154)

¼ cup red wine vinegar

PER SERVING Calories 519
Fat 34g, Protein 35g, Sodium 830mg, Total Carbs 19g, Fiber 4g

1. Preheat the oven to 400°F.

2. Season the pork with the chili powder, paprika, garlic powder, onion powder, cumin, salt, and pepper. In an ovenproof skillet over high heat, heat the ghee and sear each side of the pork, about 5 minutes total, and then pour in the chicken broth and stir well to deglaze the skillet, scraping up the browned bits from the bottom.

3. Transfer the skillet to the oven and cook for 40 to 45 minutes, or until the internal temperature of the meat is 145°F. Baste the pork once or twice with the pan juices, using a spoon to pour the juices over the pork.

4. While the pork is cooking, in a large bowl, toss to combine the broccoli noodles, carrots, and onion with the mayonnaise and red wine vinegar. Season with salt and pepper, cover, and refrigerate until the pork is done.

5. Allow the pork to rest for about 10 minutes, and then dice it and add it to the slaw. Toss to combine and serve immediately.

VARIATION 1 BROCCOLI NOODLE SLAW WITH PORK AND RAISINS: Add 1 cup of golden raisins to the slaw.

VARIATION 2 BROCCOLI NOODLE SLAW WITH SPIRALIZED APPLES AND PORK: Add 1 or 2 spiralized apples to the slaw. You may need to add another tablespoon each of Paleo Mayo and red wine vinegar.

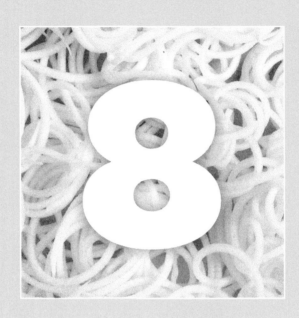

TURNIPS

I think turnips are a generally overlooked vegetable, but they have a lot to offer—they're really easy to spiralize, and they add a satisfying starchiness that makes them a great Paleo alternative to white potatoes. For a long time, I'd always reach for sweet potatoes instead of white potatoes, but I've found that turnips really do a great job imitating the carb-y comfort that makes potatoes such a staple in most diets. They're mild in flavor, so they lend themselves well to lots of different seasonings and preparation styles. This chapter includes oven-roasting, pan-frying, and even just lightly simmering.

Just a few notes about spiralizing turnips: Make sure you peel the turnips before making noodles with them—the peel is a little rough, so getting rid of that needs to be your first step. After that, turnip noodles cook quickly—just 5 to 6 minutes to soften the otherwise hard texture. Choose a small, round turnip if possible, to yield lots of long spiral noodles instead of short ones. Turnip noodles are also great when riced, so feel free to experiment!

BACON-ROASTED TURNIP NOODLES

 These bacon-roasted turnip noodles are so good and so easy to make—all you do is assemble the ingredients on a sheet pan and roast for about 15 minutes. They're a great side dish on their own, but you can easily transform this recipe into a salad by adding your favorite dressing, or add some chicken or a fried egg to turn it into a main course. I love the earthy flavor of turnips and bacon together, so this is one of my favorites. **SERVES 4**

PREP TIME: 10 minutes
COOK TIME: 10 minutes

DF **NF** **30**

2 or 3 small round turnips, peeled and spiralized

4 or 5 slices bacon, diced

1 tablespoon extra-virgin olive oil

Salt

Freshly ground black pepper

PER SERVING Calories 171 Fat 12g, Protein 9g, Sodium 842mg, Total Carbs 6g, Fiber 2g

1. Preheat the oven to 425°F.

2. On a large sheet pan, spread the turnip noodles and raw diced bacon in an even layer. Drizzle the olive oil over the noodles and season with salt and pepper.

3. Roast for 10 to 15 minutes, or until the bacon is crispy, and serve.

VARIATION 1 **PANCETTA-ROASTED TURNIP NOODLES WITH ROSEMARY:** Substitute pancetta for bacon and add 2 or 3 chopped fresh rosemary sprigs to the pan.

VARIATION 2 **BACON-ROASTED TURNIP NOODLES WITH CHICKEN:** Add about 1 pound diced cooked chicken to the cooked noodles. Toss everything to combine and serve immediately.

ONE-POT SAUSAGE and GRAVY over TURNIP NOODLES

 My mom serves her sausage and gravy over cauliflower rice, but it's excellent on top of sautéed turnip noodles, too. You can roast them for a little extra flavor, but I like sautéing them because they cook in the gravy, making this an easy one-pot recipe. Growing up in Virginia meant always having access to the very best sausage and gravy, so it's nice to have a Paleo alternative to enjoy, even if I have to skip the biscuits. **SERVES 4**

PREP TIME: 10 minutes
COOK TIME: 15 minutes

30

3 tablespoons grass-fed butter

½ yellow onion, very finely chopped

1 garlic clove, minced

1 pound pork sausage, ground

2 tablespoons arrowroot powder

½ to ¾ cup almond or coconut milk

¼ teaspoon crushed red pepper

Salt

Freshly ground black pepper

2 small round turnips, peeled and spiralized

PER SERVING Calories 591
Fat 52g, Protein 24g, Sodium 1,250mg,
Total Carbs 9g, Fiber 2g

1. In a medium skillet over medium heat, melt the butter. Sauté the onion and garlic for about 5 minutes, or until the onion becomes translucent. Add the sausage and break it up with a spoon until crumbled and starting to brown, about 5 minutes.

2. Sprinkle the arrowroot powder over the sausage and mix well to combine. Add some of the almond milk, stir, and add more if necessary—the consistency should be on the thick side.

3. Add the crushed red pepper, salt, and black pepper. Give it a stir and add the turnip noodles. Cook for 3 to 5 minutes, or until the noodles are fork-tender. Serve immediately.

VARIATION 1 ONE-POT SAUSAGE AND GRAVY OVER TURNIP NOODLES WITH MUSHROOMS: Add 10 ounces sliced mushrooms before you cook the sausage. You might need a little extra almond milk to get the right consistency. Follow the rest of the recipe as written.

VARIATION 2 ONE-POT SAUSAGE AND GRAVY OVER TURNIP NOODLES WITH SPINACH: Add 2 or 3 handfuls of fresh spinach a few minutes before serving.

TURNIP CURLY FRIES

  I like to bake my veggie curly fries because it's a little easier, but sometimes I'm really in the mood for actual *fried* fries. For this recipe, turnip noodles are trimmed into curly fry–size pieces and then fried in a shallow pan with ghee. Ghee is clarified butter with a high smoke point, so it's ideal for frying veggies. Plus, it's absolutely delicious and adds a great nutty quality to the dish. **SERVES 4**

PREP TIME: 10 minutes
COOK TIME: 10 minutes

NF **30**

3 tablespoons ghee

2 or 3 small round turnips, peeled, spiralized, and trimmed

Salt

Freshly ground black pepper

PER SERVING Calories 110 Fat 10g, Protein <1g, Sodium 351mg, Total Carbs 6g, Fiber 2g

1. In a large skillet over medium-high heat, heat the ghee. Working in batches, add the turnip fries and sauté for 5 to 7 minutes, or until they start to brown. Season with salt and pepper.

2. Transfer the fries from the skillet to a paper towel-lined plate, repeat with the remaining noodles, and serve.

VARIATION 1 **TRUFFLE OIL TURNIP CURLY FRIES:** If you're feeling a little indulgent, drizzle a very small amount (2 teaspoons or less) of truffle oil over the cooked turnip fries. Finish with a garnish of chopped parsley.

VARIATION 2 **CAJUN TURNIP CURLY FRIES:** Immediately after cooking, season the fries with 1 tablespoon Cajun seasoning (make it yourself if you can't find it: salt, garlic powder, ground paprika, freshly ground black pepper, onion powder, ground cayenne pepper, dried oregano, dried thyme, and crushed red pepper flakes).

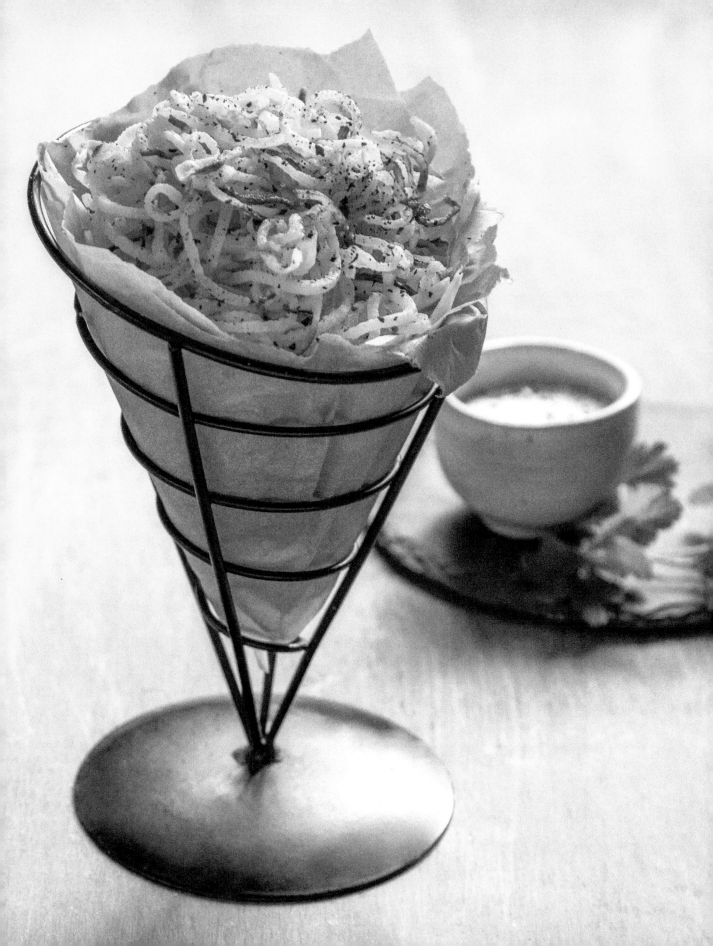

TURNIP PASTA with RED BELL PEPPER SAUCE and CHICKEN

 This creamy roasted red bell pepper sauce is really tasty, and while it takes a bit longer to make than most of the other recipes you'll find in this book, I think it's worth every minute. Apart from a blender and a small broiler pan, all you really need is one skillet. Despite the number of steps, I always appreciate a recipe that uses a minimum amount of dishware!

SERVES 4

PREP TIME: 15 minutes
COOK TIME: 35 minutes, plus 30 minutes to cool

NF

2 red bell peppers

2 tablespoons extra-virgin olive oil

2 garlic cloves, minced

1 (14.5-ounce) can coconut milk

4 tablespoons grass-fed butter, divided

Salt

Freshly ground black pepper

¼ teaspoon crushed red pepper

1½ pounds boneless chicken breasts, sliced

2 small round turnips, peeled and spiralized

¼ cup chopped fresh basil

PER SERVING Calories 761 Fat 56g, Protein 53g, Sodium 576mg, Total Carbs 15g, Fiber 4g

1. Preheat the broiler to high.

2. On a small broiler pan, lightly coat the peppers in a little bit of the olive oil. Once the broiler is ready, grill the peppers under the broiler until the skin is blackened, about 10 minutes. Put them in a plastic bag to sweat for 30 to 45 minutes.

3. Take the peppers out of the bag, peel the skin off, and remove the stem, ribs, and seeds.

4. In a large skillet over medium-high heat, sauté the garlic and roasted red peppers in the remaining olive oil for about 10 minutes, stirring frequently.

5. Carefully transfer the pepper mixture to a blender and purée. Return to the skillet over medium heat, add the coconut milk and 3 tablespoons of butter, and stir until just combined. Season with salt and pepper and add the crushed red pepper. Remove the sauce from the skillet and set aside.

6. In the same skillet over medium heat, cook the chicken in the last tablespoon of butter until cooked through, 8 to 10 minutes. Remove the chicken and add the turnip noodles to the pan. Cook the noodles for 4 to 5 minutes, or until the noodles start to become fork-tender, and then return the chicken to the pan.

7. Pour the sauce over everything, and bring to a simmer. Remove from the heat, garnish with the chopped basil, and serve immediately.

VARIATION 1 ZUCCHINI NOODLES WITH RED BELL PEPPER SAUCE AND CHICKEN: Instead of turnip noodles, use zucchini noodles for this recipe (any blade will be great) and follow the recipe as written.

VARIATION 2 TURNIP NOODLES WITH RED BELL PEPPER SAUCE AND SHRIMP: Use 1½ pounds shrimp instead of chicken breast—just cook for 2 to 3 minutes per side, or until shrimp is pink and opaque.

CHILI with TURNIP NOODLES

Lately I've been serving veggie noodles with my chilis and stews—it's a great way to use up vegetables that need to be cooked before they go bad, and spiralizing them always makes me feel like I'm having a pasta dish. This technique for this recipe is similar to my Fettuccini Bolognese (page 30) with zucchini noodles, but I love adding the zesty chili spices and serving it with a generous serving of turnip noodles. **SERVES 6**

PREP TIME: 15 minutes
COOK TIME: 3 hours, 15 minutes

DF **NF**

2 tablespoons extra-virgin olive oil

2 small round turnips, peeled and spiralized

1 large yellow onion, diced

2 or 3 garlic cloves, chopped

1 medium red bell pepper, chopped

2 pounds ground beef

1 (28-ounce) can crushed tomatoes (no sugar added)

1½ teaspoons crushed red pepper

1 tablespoon chili powder

½ teaspoon dried oregano

¾ teaspoon dry mustard

¾ teaspoon ground coriander

½ teaspoon ground allspice

1 teaspoon ground cumin

1 teaspoon ground paprika

About 2 cups chicken broth

1½ teaspoons ground cayenne pepper (more or less depending on your heat preference)

½ cup apple cider vinegar

2 or 3 green onions, finely chopped

1. In a large cast iron pot or Dutch oven over medium heat, add the olive oil and sauté the turnip noodles for about 5 minutes, or until they've softened a bit. Remove the noodles from the pot and set aside.

2. Sauté the onion, garlic, and bell peppers until tender, about 5 minutes. Add the ground beef and allow it to brown. Stir with a wooden spoon and break up the larger pieces.

3. After the beef is mostly browned, about 5 minutes, add the canned tomatoes. Give it a good stir and add the crushed red pepper, chili powder, oregano, dry mustard, coriander, allspice, cumin, and paprika.

4. Bring the chili to a low boil, and then reduce the heat to low and simmer for 2 to 3 hours. Periodically add chicken broth and stir when it starts getting thick.

5. About 20 minutes before serving, add the cayenne pepper and apple cider vinegar. To serve, fill bowls with the turnip noodles, spoon the chili over them, and garnish with the sliced green onions.

PER SERVING Calories 438, Fat 15g, Protein 52g, Sodium 665mg, Total Carbs 21g, Fiber 7g

VARIATION 1 CHICKEN CHILI WITH TURNIP NOODLES: Use ground chicken instead of beef for a chicken chili.

VARIATION 2 BEEF AND PORK CHILI WITH TURNIP NOODLES: Add more flavor to this dish by using half ground beef and half ground pork. You can also switch the chicken broth to beef broth. Make this chili ahead of time by cooking it in a slow cooker for 8 hours on low. For improved flavor, sauté the vegetables and brown the meat ahead of time and then add the rest of the ingredients.

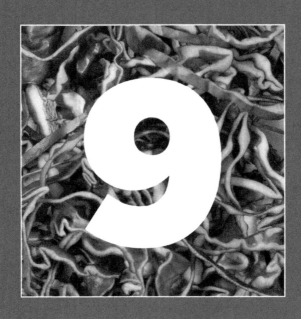

9

CABBAGE

I love cabbage because it lends itself well to a ton of different flavors, and it's tender enough to eat raw but stands up to cooking as well. It also lasts forever in the fridge, so you can leave it whole (I like picking the leaves off a few at a time and using them as Paleo wraps for turkey and vegetables at lunchtime), or you can spiralize it and use it immediately or store for a few more days.

Note: When spiralizing, remove the outside layers until you have a tight ball of leaves that aren't sticking out—the outside layers won't cooperate with the spiralizer, so it's best to just remove them and use them for something else.

KIMCHI CABBAGE NOODLES

 Kimchi is a staple in Korean kitchens, and while it can seem a bit intimidating to make yourself, it's really quite easy. Because it's a fermented product, you do have to let it sit at room temperature for a few days, so if that's not your thing, I've included a quick pickled variation. I love kimchi—it offers a nice spicy bite to just about everything, although I've been known to eat it straight out of the jar, too. **SERVES 6**

PREP TIME: 20 minutes, plus 5 days to ferment

1 large napa cabbage, spiralized

¼ cup kosher salt

2 or 3 garlic cloves, minced

1 (2-inch) piece peeled fresh ginger, sliced (about 2 tablespoons)

¼ cup fish sauce

1 to 4 tablespoons gochugaru—Korean red pepper powder (depending on your heat preference)

2 or 3 carrots, sliced

1 daikon radish, sliced thin

PER SERVING Calories 109 Fat 2g, Protein 4g, Sodium 1,486mg, Total Carbs 20g, Fiber 4g

1. In a large bowl, sprinkle the salt over the cabbage. Massage the cabbage noodles with your hands for a few minutes, until they start to wilt slightly. Add enough water to the bowl to cover the cabbage, and cover with a plate weighed down with a couple of cans—you want to put some pressure on the cabbage. Let it rest like that for 1 to 2 hours.

2. Rinse the cabbage well and drain it in a colander for 10 to 15 minutes. Squeeze the cabbage to remove any leftover water, return the cabbage to the bowl and add the garlic, ginger, fish sauce, and gochugaru. Add the carrots and daikon and mix thoroughly. Pack the kimchi into clean, dry canning jars. Press down until the brine covers the cabbage, leaving about 1 inch of space at the top of the jar.

3. Cover loosely and store on your counter for 1 to 5 days, checking daily for flavor preference. The mixture may bubble over—keeping the jars in a pie plate or other rimmed vessel will contain any spillover during the fermentation process. When it's "ripe" enough for your liking, transfer to the refrigerator.

VARIATION 1 QUICK-PICKLED KIMCHI: Boil 5 cups water with ½ cup kosher salt. Let it cool slightly. In a large bowl, pour the brine over the cabbage noodles. Soak the cabbage for about 15 minutes, stirring once halfway through. Rinse and drain the cabbage as directed in the original recipe. Combine the garlic, ginger, fish sauce, and gochugaru and mix with the carrots, daikon, and drained cabbage. Pack into jars and refrigerate immediately. Enjoy within 5 to 10 days.

VARIATION 2 KIMCHI WITH CUCUMBERS: Add 1 sliced or spiralized cucumber to either of the above recipes.

CABBAGE SOUP

Cabbage soup gets a bad rep for being bland and boring, but if it's seasoned properly, it can be a delicious and comforting classic that's both budget-friendly and filling. I like to make mine with beef broth for an even richer flavor, but you could easily swap that out for chicken or veggie, depending on your preferences and/or what you have on hand. **SERVES 6**

PREP TIME: 10 minutes
COOK TIME: 25 minutes

NF

3 tablespoons grass-fed butter

1 medium yellow onion, diced

2 carrots, diced

2 celery stalks, diced

1 garlic clove, minced

1 large cabbage, spiralized

1 (14-ounce) can diced tomatoes

4 to 5 cups beef broth

1 dried bay leaf

Salt

Freshly ground black pepper

Fresh parsley sprigs, for garnish

PER SERVING Calories 121 Fat 7g, Protein 6g, Sodium 706mg, Total Carbs 9g, Fiber 3g

1. In a large saucepan over medium heat, melt the butter. Sauté the onion for about 5 minutes, until translucent. Add the carrots and celery and cook for another 4 to 5 minutes, or until the veggies become fork-tender. Add the garlic and cabbage noodles. Stir to combine and continue to cook over medium heat.

2. Add the can of tomatoes (and any liquid) to the pot and stir. Pour the beef broth in and bring to a simmer. Add the bay leaf and reduce the heat to low, cooking for another 10 to 15 minutes.

3. Season with salt and pepper and serve with a sprinkle of fresh parsley.

VARIATION 1 CHICKEN AND CABBAGE SOUP: Once the broth is simmering, add about 1 pound boneless, skinless chicken thighs or breasts to the pot and poach until cooked through, about 10 minutes. Remove the chicken from the broth, shred it, and return it to the saucepan. If you have some leftover cooked chicken on hand, just stir it into the soup a few minutes before serving and simmer until heated through.

VARIATION 2 CABBAGE AND ZUCCHINI NOODLE SOUP: Add more veggies to this soup (and get rid of any leftover zoodles you may have in your fridge) by adding 1 or 2 spiralized zucchini to the pot 2 to 3 minutes before you're ready to serve.

ASIAN PURPLE CABBAGE NOODLE SLAW

 This Asian-inspired cabbage noodle slaw is delicious on its own or paired with shrimp or beef. I love purple cabbage because it has such a nice crunch and a heartier texture than other cabbages. The spicy sesame-lime dressing is easy to customize if you don't like spicy food, and it's super good on other salads and slaws, or even chicken. **SERVES 6**

PREP TIME: 10 minutes

DF NF R 30

Juice of 2 limes

3 tablespoons sesame oil

1 tablespoon coconut aminos

1 teaspoon chili garlic oil

1 tablespoon honey (optional)

Salt

Freshly ground black pepper

1 large purple cabbage (also referred to as red cabbage), spiralized

1 or 2 green onions, finely chopped

2 tablespoons sesame seeds

PER SERVING Calories 109 Fat 9g, Protein 1g, Sodium 303mg, Total Carbs 6g, Fiber 1g

1. In a small bowl, mix to combine the lime juice, sesame oil, coconut aminos, chili garlic oil, and honey (if using). Season with salt and pepper.

2. In a large bowl, toss to combine the cabbage noodles and the dressing. Season with a little more salt and pepper if necessary.

3. Serve immediately with green onions and a sprinkle of sesame seeds.

VARIATION 1 ASIAN PURPLE CABBAGE NOODLE SLAW WITH AVOCADO: Serve this slaw topped with ½ sliced avocado.

VARIATION 2 CREAMY PURPLE CABBAGE NOODLE ASIAN SLAW: Make this dressing creamy by adding 1 to 2 tablespoons tahini. Mix well to combine.

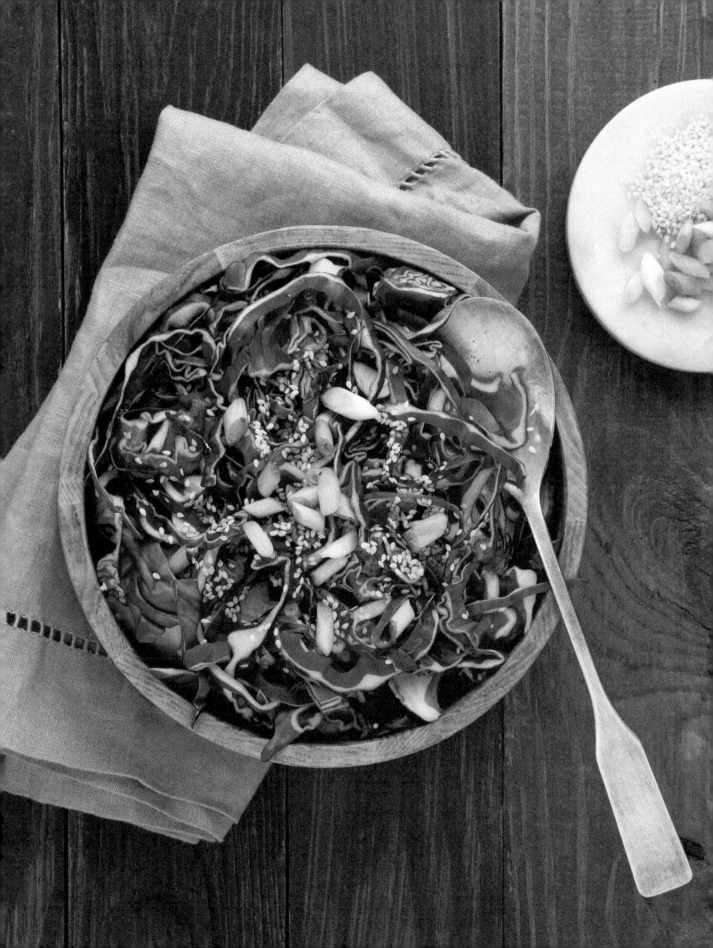

PALEO CABBAGE SLAW

 My mom makes this cabbage slaw all the time. It's delicious, but it's always a big pain to make because chopping cabbage can make a huge mess. That's one convenient thing about having a spiralizer—even if you aren't making a special spiralized recipe, you can easily use it to slice and chop vegetables, especially big ones like cabbage or onions. This recipe is exactly the way Mom makes it, only it's made quicker by spiralizing the cabbage into noodles instead of chopping everything up by hand. **SERVES 6**

PREP TIME: 10 minutes, plus 15 minutes to chill

1 cup Paleo Mayo (page 154)

2 to 3 tablespoons agave

2 tablespoons apple cider vinegar

2 teaspoons celery seed

Salt

Freshly ground black pepper

1 small to medium cabbage, spiralized

PER SERVING Calories 194 Fat 13g, Protein <1g, Sodium 478mg, Total Carbs 20g, Fiber <1g

1. In a small bowl, combine the mayonnaise, agave, apple cider vinegar, and celery seed. Stir well and season with salt and pepper.

2. In a large bowl, spoon the dressing over the cabbage noodles and toss to combine.

3. Refrigerate for at least 15 to 20 minutes before serving.

VARIATION 1 PALEO CABBAGE SLAW WITH SLOW-COOKED PULLED PORK: Make this side dish into a main course by adding about 1 pound pulled pork. It's easy to make pulled pork in your slow cooker: Combine pork butt, 1 to 2 cups of your favorite (sugar-free) barbecue sauce, and some salt and pepper. Cook on low for 8 hours. Plan ahead by making the pork the night before so it's ready when you are.

VARIATION 2 PALEO CARROT SLAW: Instead of cabbage, make this slaw with about 1 pound spiralized carrots.

SPICY KOREAN BEEF NOODLES

 I love cabbage noodles because they cook quickly and pair well with Asian flavors. These spicy Korean beef noodle bowls are one of my favorite things to make when I'm craving Asian food but don't want to blow my diet (or budget) with takeout. Cabbage lasts such a long time in the fridge, so I always try to have one on hand, along with chili garlic sauce and sesame oil. **SERVES 4**

PREP TIME: 10 minutes
COOK TIME: 15 minutes

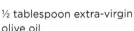

½ tablespoon extra-virgin olive oil

½ red onion, sliced thin

1 garlic clove, minced

1 pound flank steak, sliced thin

1 small to medium cabbage, spiralized (napa cabbage would be good for this)

1 to 2 teaspoons chili garlic oil or chili garlic sauce

1½ tablespoons sesame oil

1 tablespoon coconut aminos

½ large cucumber, diced, for garnish

2 or 3 green onions, chopped, for garnish

2 to 3 tablespoons chopped fresh cilantro, for garnish

PER SERVING Calories 112
Fat 9g, Protein 2g, Sodium 163mg,
Total Carbs 7g, Fiber 2g

1. In a large skillet over medium heat, heat the olive oil and sauté the red onion for about 5 minutes. Add the garlic and the steak and cook the steak pieces for about 3 minutes per side.

2. Add the cabbage to the skillet and sauté for 3 to 4 minutes, or until the cabbage noodles are beginning to wilt. Lower the heat to medium-low and add the chili garlic oil, sesame oil, and coconut aminos. Stir until combined and remove from the heat.

3. Spoon into bowls, garnish with the cucumber, green onions, and cilantro, and serve.

VARIATION 1 SPICY KOREAN BEEF NOODLES WITH SPINACH: Add 2 cups spinach to the skillet with the cabbage noodles.

VARIATION 2 VEGETARIAN SPICY KOREAN NOODLES: Skip the beef and serve these bowls topped with a fried egg. To fry eggs, crack them right into the skillet you used for the cabbage noodles, adding a little grass-fed butter if necessary, and cook on one side until the white is no longer runny. Carefully flip and cook for 1 or 2 minutes on the other side, depending on how done you want the yolk.

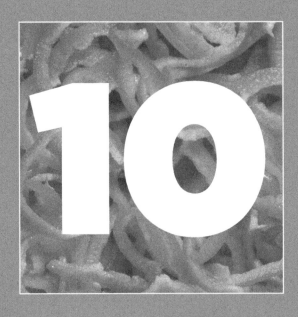

10

BELL PEPPERS

Bell pepper is another vegetable that's delicious both raw and cooked. I love spiralizing them and incorporating them in dishes with a wide variety of flavors and preparation styles. They might seem a little tricky to spiralize since they're hollow, but if you just cut the very top off, you can attach the sliced side to the handle and spiralize first, then rinse to remove any seeds that are left over.

TRI-COLOR BELL PEPPER ANTIPASTO SALAD
with OLIVES and TUNA

 I love a vinaigrette-based tuna salad with olives. The red, yellow, and green bell pepper noodles are colorful and flavorful, and also a little bit fancy, so you can make it for guests and feel good about serving a healthy, interesting meal that takes only a few minutes to throw together. You could easily marinate the tuna ahead of time and toss it with the peppers and tomatoes right before serving. **SERVES 4**

PREP TIME: 10 minutes

2 (6-ounce) cans tuna, drained

½ cup sliced black olives

¼ cup balsamic vinaigrette (see page 47)

1 green bell pepper, spiralized

1 yellow bell pepper, spiralized

1 red bell pepper, spiralized

½ cup cherry tomatoes, halved

Salt

Freshly ground black pepper

PER SERVING Calories 270 Fat 15g, Protein 24g, Sodium 603mg, Total Carbs 10g, Fiber 2g

In a large bowl, mix to combine the tuna and olives with the balsamic vinaigrette. Add the bell pepper noodles and cherry tomatoes and toss to combine. Season with salt and pepper and serve immediately.

VARIATION 1 TRI-COLOR BELL PEPPER ANTIPASTO SALAD WITH CUCUMBERS: Instead of olives, add 1 spiralized cucumber to the salad with the bell pepper noodles.

VARIATION 2 TRI-COLOR BELL PEPPER ANTIPASTO SALAD WITH LEMON VINAIGRETTE: Follow the original recipe as written, but use lemon juice instead of balsamic vinegar in the dressing.

PHILLY "NO CHEESE" STEAK LETTUCE WRAPS

BLADE

This is a Paleo take on the classic Philly cheesesteak sandwich, except that we're skipping the bread and there's no cheese—just onions, green pepper noodles, and delicious sliced steak sautéed together in the delicious combination that made the sandwich so famous. The trick to getting all the vegetables done perfectly is to give each of them their own time in the pan and then stir it all together before serving. **SERVES 4**

PREP TIME: 10 minutes
COOK TIME: 30 minutes

NF

3 tablespoons grass-fed butter, divided

1 medium yellow onion, sliced

2 garlic cloves

Salt

Freshly ground black pepper

2 green peppers, spiralized

1½ pounds steak, sliced thin

4 to 6 large romaine or butter lettuce leaves

1 to 2 tablespoons Paleo Mayo (page 154)

PER SERVING Calories 444
Fat 17g, Protein 63g, Sodium 464mg, Total Carbs 8g, Fiber 2g

1. In a large skillet over medium heat, melt 1 tablespoon of butter. Sauté the onion and garlic together, stirring regularly, and cook for longer than usual—about 10 to 15 minutes. Season with salt and pepper, remove from the skillet, and set aside.

2. Add the green pepper noodles and sauté for 8 to 10 minutes, or until the noodles start to become fork-tender. Season with salt and pepper, remove from the skillet, and set aside with the onions.

3. Add the remaining 2 tablespoons of butter and the steak to the skillet and season with salt and pepper. Cook over medium heat until the meat browns. Return the onions and green peppers to the skillet and stir over medium-high heat for 2 to 3 minutes.

4. To assemble the lettuce wraps, place lettuce leaves on a plate and add some of the steak and veggie mixture to each. Add a dollop of mayonnaise and enjoy immediately.

VARIATION 1 PHILLY "NO CHEESE" STEAK LETTUCE WRAPS WITH MUSHROOMS: Add about 10 ounces sliced mushrooms to this recipe—sauté separately in a little butter for 6 to 7 minutes, or until browned and beginning to crisp around the edges, before following the remaining recipe steps as written.

VARIATION 2 PHILLY "NO CHEESE" STEAK OMELET: Instead of making lettuce wraps with the steak, green pepper, and onion mixture, make it into an omelet—after removing all the sautéed items from the skillet, add 2 or 3 whisked eggs to the skillet along with a little grass-fed butter, if necessary. Let the eggs spread out and cook on one side, then flip gently before adding all the filling back to the pan. Fold the eggs over the filling and serve hot.

CHICKEN FAJITA SKILLET

 Is there anything better than a sizzling platter of fajitas? Chicken fajitas are always my go-to order whenever I'm out somewhere that serves Mexican food—it's easy to customize it to be Paleo without abandoning the main components of the dish. I just ask for fajitas without tortillas, rice, beans, or cheese—sometimes they'll even give you a little extra avocado to make up for it. I like to make this chicken fajita skillet and eat it on its own, since it's full of veggies and meat, but you could also put it over a salad if you have any leftovers. **SERVES 4**

PREP TIME: 10 minutes
COOK TIME: 15 minutes

2 tablespoons extra-virgin olive oil

½ yellow onion, diced

2 or 3 garlic cloves, minced

1 green bell pepper, spiralized

1 red bell pepper, spiralized

1 orange bell pepper, spiralized

1½ pounds boneless, skinless chicken breast, diced

2 tablespoons Taco Seasoning (page 155)

Salt

Freshly ground black pepper

PER SERVING Calories 172
Fat 10g, Protein 11g, Sodium 360mg,
Total Carbs 11g, Fiber 3g

1. In a large ovenproof skillet over medium heat, heat the olive oil and sauté the onion and garlic together. After about 5 minutes, add the bell pepper noodles. Stir everything together and cook over medium-high heat for 3 to 4 minutes, or until the noodles start to become fork-tender.

2. Add the diced chicken and taco seasoning and cook for 6 to 8 minutes, until all sides are browned and the chicken is cooked through. Season with salt and pepper and serve hot.

VARIATION 1 **CHICKEN FAJITA SKILLET WITH AVOCADO:** Top each serving with ½ diced avocado and a wedge of lime, for garnish.

VARIATION 2 **STEAK AND SHRIMP FAJITA SKILLET:** Instead of chicken, sauté ½ pound shrimp and 1 pound sliced steak in the skillet for 5 to 6 minutes, or until the steak is mostly cooked through. Follow the remaining recipe steps as written.

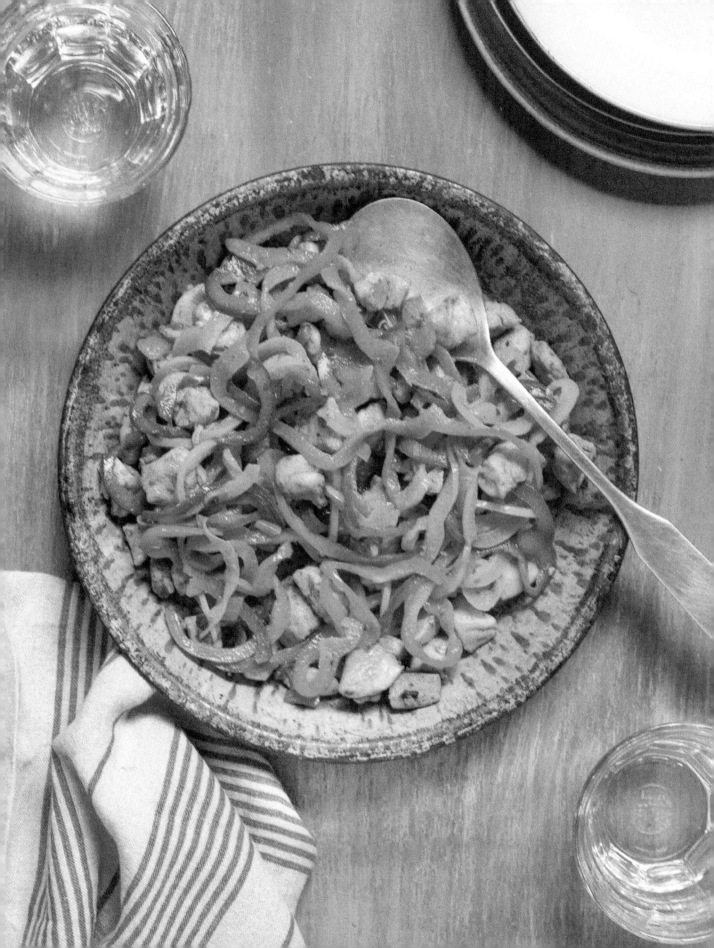

EMPANADA GREEN PEPPER NOODLES

 My mom is from Argentina, so growing up we always had empanadas at home. They were my favorite, and the recipe has kind of become a tradition in our family. Now that we eat Paleo, we just skip the dumpling dough that traditionally holds it all together, but we still make the filling and eat it with eggs, salads, and even on its own, as in this recipe. **SERVES 4**

PREP TIME: 10 minutes
COOK TIME: 15 minutes

1 tablespoon extra-virgin olive oil

1 medium yellow onion, diced

2 garlic cloves, minced

1 pound ground beef

1 cup sliced green olives

2 green peppers, spiralized

2 hard-boiled eggs, diced

Salt

Freshly ground black pepper

PER SERVING Calories 336
Fat 17g, Protein 38g, Sodium 692mg,
Total Carbs 8g, Fiber 3g

1. In a large skillet over medium heat, heat the olive oil and sauté the onion and garlic. After about 5 minutes, add the ground beef and stir everything together for about 3 minutes more.

2. Add the sliced olives and green pepper noodles. Sauté for another 3 to 4 minutes, or until the noodles start to become fork-tender, add the diced eggs and season with salt and pepper. Remove from the heat and serve immediately.

VARIATION 1 EMPANADA GREEN PEPPER NOODLES WITH TURKEY: Use ground turkey instead of beef if you want to lighten this recipe up a bit.

VARIATION 2 EMPANADA GREEN PEPPER AND CARROT NOODLES: Add 2 or 3 spiralized carrots (blade D) to the skillet with the green peppers.

ITALIAN SAUSAGES with BELL PEPPER NOODLES

 One of the easiest meals you can throw together is just sautéed onions and peppers with Italian sausages, and people always seem to love it. This recipe uses bell pepper noodles instead of chopped bell peppers, which saves a lot of prep time and makes eating a little more fun. I like making this dish because once you cut your onion and spiralize the peppers, all you have to do is add sausage and throw it in the oven. **SERVES 4**

PREP TIME: 10 minutes
COOK TIME: 20 minutes

DF **NF**

3 green bell peppers, spiralized

1 medium yellow onion, sliced

2 tablespoons extra-virgin olive oil

Salt

Freshly ground black pepper

½ teaspoon garlic powder

2 pounds whole spicy Italian sausage

PER SERVING Calories 870 Fat 72g, Protein 45g, Sodium 1,993mg, Total Carbs 10g, Fiber 2g

1. Preheat the oven to 425°F.

2. Add the bell pepper noodles and sliced onion to a large baking dish. Drizzle the olive oil over the vegetables and season with salt, pepper, and garlic powder. Add the sausages to the dish, arranging them evenly next to one another.

3. Bake for 20 to 30 minutes, or until the sausages are cooked through, and serve.

VARIATION 1 ITALIAN SAUSAGE WITH BELL PEPPER NOODLES AND MUSHROOMS: Add about 10 ounces sliced mushrooms to the dish with the other vegetables.

VARIATION 2 BAKED CHICKEN THIGHS WITH BELL PEPPER NOODLES: Instead of Italian sausages, add 2 pounds chicken thighs to the baking dish. Season with salt and pepper and about ¼ teaspoon crushed red pepper.

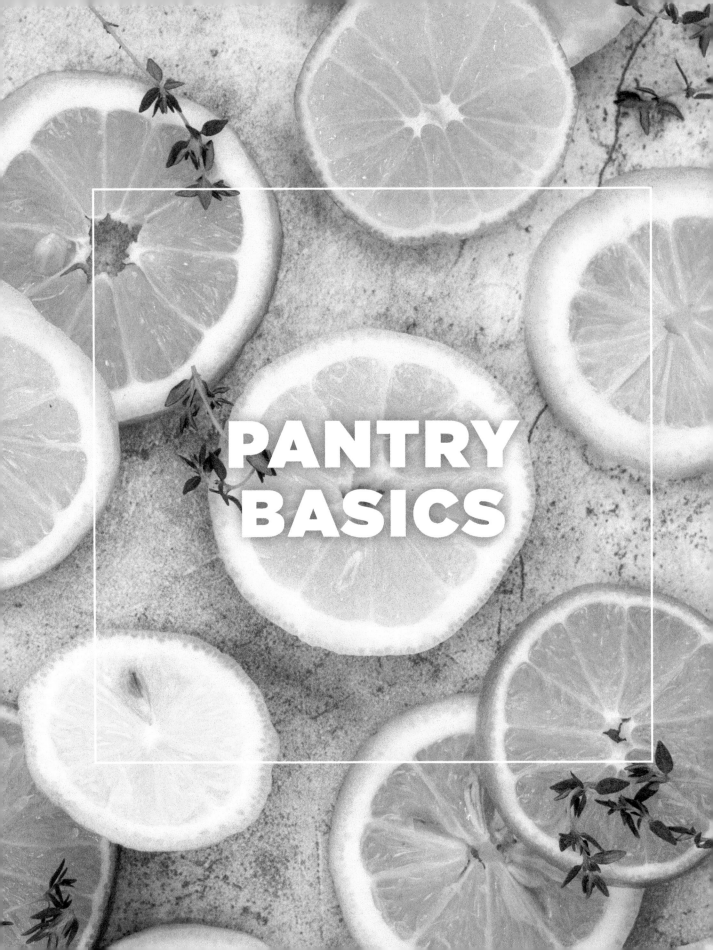

PANTRY BASICS

The Paleo pantry is somewhat of an enigma—what sauces and dips are Paleo, which aren't? The short answer is that pretty much nothing you can buy premade in a bottle is Paleo, but that doesn't mean you can't easily make Paleo versions of your favorite sauces and snacks. This chapter covers just a few dipping sauces, seasonings, and snacks that usually contain sugar or some other non-Paleo additive.

PALEO MAYO
(and Paleo Ranch Dressing)

The following two recipes are in my first book, but I wanted to include them here as well because I use them in a lot of these new recipes, too. Homemade mayo really is the only Paleo mayo out there, and I love whipping up a batch of Paleo Ranch Dressing every week for salads and quick veggie platter snacks.

MAKES 1¼ CUPS

PREP TIME: 10 minutes, plus 20 minutes to bring to room temperature

1 egg, at room temperature

2 tablespoons freshly squeezed lemon juice, at room temperature

½ teaspoon salt

1 teaspoon dried mustard

1¼ cups extra-virgin olive oil, divided

1. In a food processor, add the egg, lemon juice, salt, dried mustard, and ¼ cup of olive oil and quickly process to combine.

2. With the food processor still running, slowly drizzle in the remaining 1 cup of olive oil. When you have about 2 tablespoons of oil left, pour it in quickly.

3. Keep the mayo refrigerated until the expiration date on the eggs you use—you may wish to make a note on the container to help you remember.

VARIATION **PALEO RANCH DRESSING:** It's easy to turn your mayo into delicious ranch dressing! Add ½ cup coconut milk, ½ tablespoon dried chives, 1 teaspoon dried mustard, ½ teaspoon dried dill, ½ teaspoon celery seed, ½ teaspoon garlic powder, and ½ teaspoon onion powder to 1 cup of Paleo Mayo and season with salt and pepper. Mix well and store in the fridge in an airtight container.

PER SERVING (2 tablespoons) Calories 225, Fat 26g, Protein <1g, Sodium 123mg, Total Carbs <1g, Fiber 0g

GARLIC AIOLI

I don't know about you, but my favorite thing to dip a French fry in isn't ketchup, but mayonnaise—especially if that mayonnaise is seasoned with garlic or truffle oil (or anything, really). This garlic aioli is super easy to make and will be delicious with your spiralized sweet potato, turnip, or carrot fries. **MAKES 1 CUP**

PREP TIME: 5 minutes
COOK TIME: 40 minutes

1 head garlic

1 tablespoon extra-virgin olive oil

1 cup Paleo Mayo (page 154)

Salt

Freshly ground black pepper

1. Preheat the oven to 350°F.

2. To roast the garlic, cut off the top, drizzle with the olive oil, and wrap in foil. Bake for about 40 minutes.

3. Remove from the oven, cool slightly, and then pop the cloves out of the skin. In a food processor, process to combine the garlic cloves with the mayonnaise. Season with salt and pepper and store in fridge until ready to serve.

PER SERVING (2 tablespoons) Calories 135, Fat 12g, Protein <1g, Sodium 357mg, Total Carbs 8g, Fiber 0g

TACO SEASONING

I like making my own taco seasoning because I recently realized that I usually have all the ingredients that go into it on hand, and if there's one thing I hate, it's buying something that I can make myself. If you have a reasonably stocked spice cabinet, I bet you can make it yourself, too—and you don't have to check labels for additives or sugar anymore!

MAKES 3 TABLESPOONS

PREP TIME: 5 minutes

1½ teaspoons ground cumin

1 tablespoon chili powder

1 teaspoon salt

1 teaspoon freshly ground black pepper

½ teaspoon ground paprika

¼ teaspoon garlic powder

¼ teaspoon onion powder

¼ to ½ teaspoon crushed red pepper flakes (depending on your heat preference)

¼ teaspoon dried oregano

In an airtight container with a lid, mix together the cumin, chili powder, salt, black pepper, paprika, garlic powder, onion powder, red pepper flakes, and oregano. Store in the airtight container.

PER SERVING (1 tablespoon) Calories 17, Fat <1g, Protein <1g, Sodium 803mg, Total Carbs 3g, Fiber 1g

ENCHILADA SAUCE

Even more so than with taco seasoning, I like to make my own enchilada sauce because the canned ones, while convenient and delicious, are often full of non-Paleo oils, sugars, and sometimes even flour. You'll need a batch of this sauce for my Chicken Enchilada Noodle Bake (page 97), but I also like it over chicken and veggies in a skillet when I'm in the mood for Mexican food but want to make something quick and healthy. **MAKES 2 ½ CUPS**

PREP TIME: 5 minutes
COOK TIME: 10 to 15 minutes

¼ cup extra-virgin olive oil

2 garlic cloves, grated

½ medium yellow onion, grated

1 (8-ounce) can plain tomato sauce (no sugar added)

½ teaspoon ground cumin

3 tablespoons chili powder

Salt

Freshly ground black pepper

1 cup chicken broth or water, if needed

1. In a large skillet over medium heat, heat the olive oil and sauté the garlic and onion for about 5 minutes, until translucent.

2. Add the tomato sauce, cumin, chili powder, salt, and pepper. Bring to a low boil and reduce the heat to simmer. Reduce until thickened, adding a little chicken broth at a time if it gets too thick.

PER SERVING (½ cup) Calories 126, Fat 11g, Protein 2g, Sodium 669mg, Total Carbs 7g, Fiber 3g

SPIRALIZED QUICK-PICKLED ONIONS

I love pickled red onions on almost anything—and they're so easy to make! I serve them with burgers and on top of salads and often just eat them on their own. Spiralizing an onion is so much quicker and easier than slicing or dicing it, so these quick-pickled onion noodles are a favorite. **SERVES 6**

PREP TIME: 5 minutes
COOK TIME: 10 minutes, plus 2 hours to cool

½ cup apple cider or rice vinegar

½ cup water

¼ cup honey

1 tablespoon salt

1 tablespoon black peppercorns

1 tablespoon mustard seeds

1 red onion, spiralized

1. In a small pot over high heat, bring the vinegar, water, honey, salt, peppercorns, and mustard seeds to a boil. Remove from the heat.

2. Pack the onion noodles into jars and pour the brine over them. Allow to cool to room temperature before covering and refrigerating for at least 2 hours.

PER SERVING Calories 31, Fat 0g, Protein 0g, Sodium 389mg, Total Carbs 8g, Fiber 0g

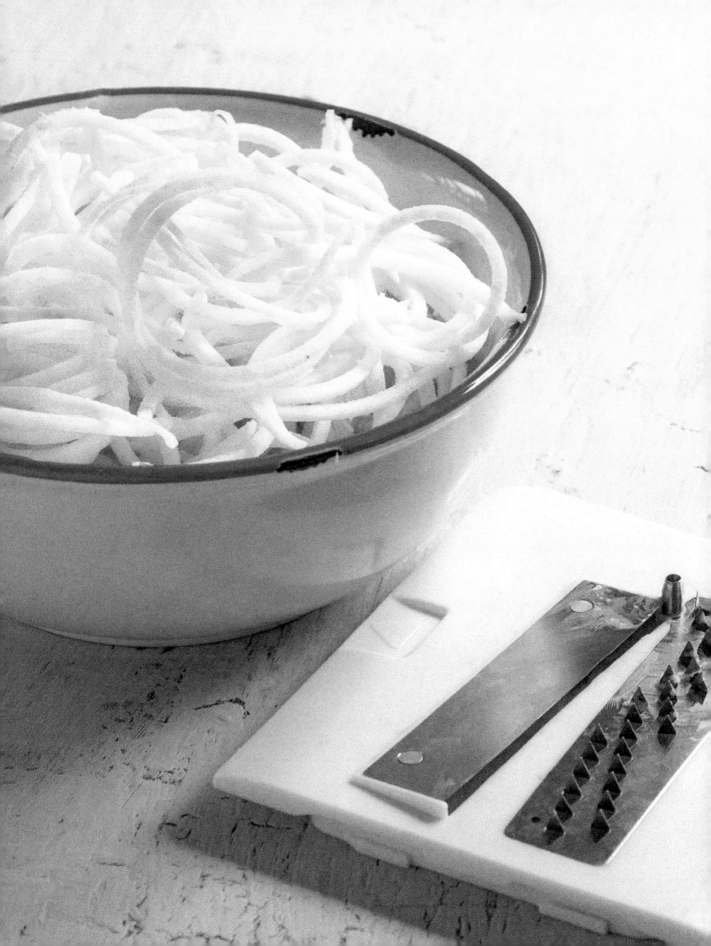

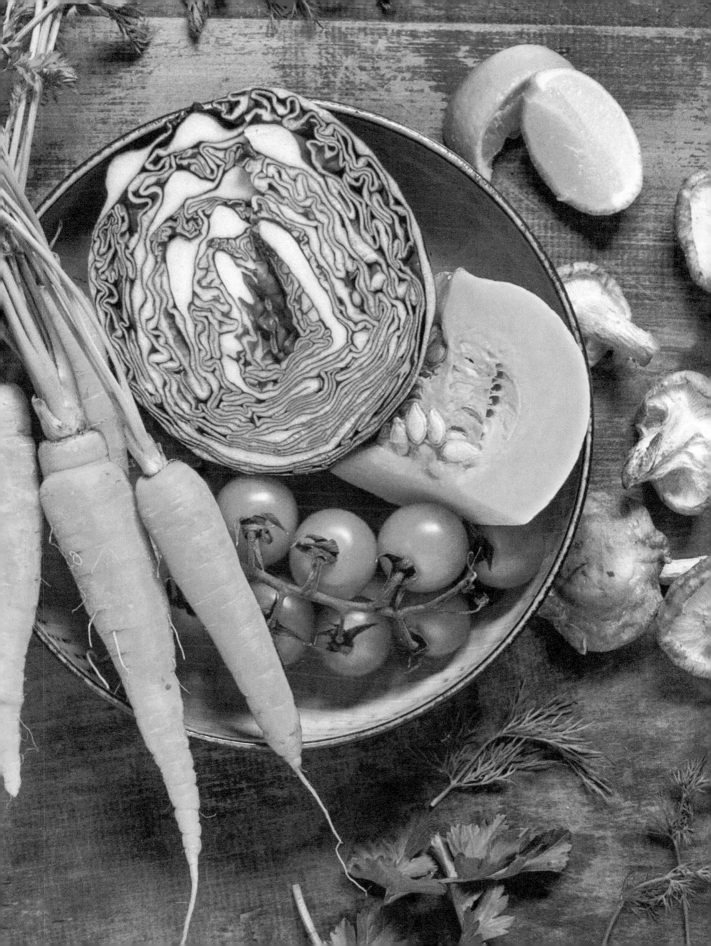

The Dirty Dozen and the Clean Fifteen

A nonprofit environmental watchdog organization called Environmental Working Group (EWG) looks at data supplied by the U.S. Department of Agriculture (USDA) and the Food and Drug Administration (FDA) about pesticide residues. Each year it compiles a list of the best and worst pesticide loads found in commercial crops. You can use these lists to decide which fruits and vegetables to buy organic to minimize your exposure to pesticides and which produce is considered safe enough to buy conventionally. This does not mean they are pesticide-free, though, so wash these fruits and vegetables thoroughly.

DIRTY DOZEN

Apples
Celery
Cherry tomatoes
Cucumbers
Grapes
Nectarines (imported)
Peaches
Potatoes
Snap peas (imported)
Spinach
Strawberries
Sweet bell peppers

In addition to the Dirty Dozen, the EWG added two types of produce contaminated with highly toxic organophosphate insecticides:

Kale/collard greens   Hot peppers

CLEAN FIFTEEN

Asparagus
Avocados
Cabbage
Cantaloupes (domestic)
Cauliflower
Eggplants
Grapefruits
Kiwis
Mangoes
Onions
Papayas
Pineapples
Sweet corn
Sweet peas (frozen)
Sweet potatoes

Measurements and Conversion Tables

VOLUME EQUIVALENTS (LIQUID)

US STANDARD	US STANDARD (OUNCES)	METRIC (APPROXIMATE)
2 tablespoons	1 fl. oz.	30 mL
¼ cup	2 fl. oz.	60 mL
½ cup	4 fl. oz.	120 mL
1 cup	8 fl. oz.	240 mL
1½ cups	12 fl. oz.	355 mL
2 cups or 1 pint	16 fl. oz.	475 mL
4 cups or 1 quart	32 fl. oz.	1 L
1 gallon	128 fl. oz.	4 L

OVEN TEMPERATURES

FAHRENHEIT (F)	CELSIUS (C) (APPROXIMATE)
250°	120°
300°	150°
325°	165°
350°	180°
375°	190°
400°	200°
425°	220°
450°	230°

VOLUME EQUIVALENTS (DRY)

US STANDARD	METRIC (APPROXIMATE)
⅛ teaspoon	0.5 mL
¼ teaspoon	1 mL
½ teaspoon	2 mL
¾ teaspoon	4 mL
1 teaspoon	5 mL
1 tablespoon	15 mL
¼ cup	59 mL
⅓ cup	79 mL
½ cup	118 mL
⅔ cup	156 mL
¾ cup	177 mL
1 cup	235 mL
2 cups or 1 pint	475 mL
3 cups	700 mL
4 cups or 1 quart	1 L

WEIGHT EQUIVALENTS

US STANDARD	METRIC (APPROXIMATE)
½ ounce	15 g
1 ounce	30 g
2 ounces	60 g
4 ounces	115 g
8 ounces	225 g
12 ounces	340 g
16 ounces or 1 pound	455 g

Resources

- **Paderno 4-Blade Spiralizer**
  www.padernousa.com/4-blade-spiralizer/
  This is the first spiralizer that I ever heard of—before this I was slicing my veggie noodles with a potato peeler!

- **The Inspiralizer**
  inspiralized.com/the-inspiralizer/
  This is the spiralizer I use. I'm a big fan of it, and it's not so big that it takes up too much room on my counter. (I use it so much that I never really put it away.)

- **KitchenAid Spiralizer Attachment**
  www.kitchenaid.com/shop/ -[KSM1APC]-5505597/KSM1APC/#
  If you're weary of purchasing another gadget for your kitchen but you own a KitchenAid mixer, you can get a spiralizer attachment for it! It's a little pricy, but I've heard nothing but good reviews. My best friend Tina has one and says she loves it.

- **Veggetti**
  buyveggetti.com/
  The Veggetti is a hand-held spiralizer that I started out with before upgrading to a countertop model—if you're not interested in committing to a full spiralizer, this small, manual one can be a really good place to start (but you won't be able to choose a noodle shape or spiralize some of the larger vegetables in this book).

- **The Big 15 Paleo Cookbook**
  bit.ly/big-15-paleo-cookbook
  This is my first cookbook, and while it only has a handful of veggie noodle recipes, it's a great place to start if you're looking for more Paleo recipes.

- **Whole 30**
  whole30.com/
  I've never done a Whole 30 but do think it can be a great place to start if you're feeling unsure or overwhelmed about changing your diet. The community is great and has lots of meal ideas and inspiration on the site, as well as their Instagram feeds (@whole30 and @whole30recipes).

- **Paleo Subreddit**
  www.reddit.com/r/paleo
  A great forum for sharing stories and asking questions. I was on here all the time when I first started out. Take everything with a grain of salt—most advice you will encounter is through experience and not necessarily expertise, but I have always found it really helpful.

Label Index

Recipe Index

General Index

180

Acknowledgments

Many thanks go to my family, who believes in me to no end. You make me feel like I can do anything.

Thank you again to Callisto Media for giving me the opportunity to write another book. It is such a pleasure working with all of you.

To my readers—of both the blog and my cookbooks—I thank you. My life and career would not be the same if you weren't in them. Thank you for your support, your feedback, and your love. It means the world to me.

Thanks to my beautiful and smart and successful friends, Corri and Haley, for pushing me to work harder every day. You're both an inspiration, and I don't think you know how much either of you mean to me.

And to my husband, Rob, thank you for being my rock when things get crazy. I know our life isn't always what we planned, but I love our adventures and wouldn't be following this path with anyone else. Thank you—I love you.

About the Author

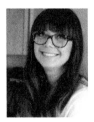

Megan Flynn Peterson is the writer behind *Freckled Italian*, a blog that focuses on life, love, personal style, nostalgia, and lots of food. She has called Virginia, Minnesota, and North Carolina home but currently resides in the San Francisco Bay Area with her husband and their rescue pup. This is her second cookbook.

You can read more from Megan at freckleditalian.com/blog, or find her on Instagram and Twitter @mflynnpete.

CPSIA information can be obtained
at www.ICGtesting.com
Printed in the USA
BVOW11s1506020417
479923BV00002B/2/P